I0121141

Dorset's Private Asylums

Dedicated to my children, Ben and Kate,
and my parents, May and Peter

Dorset's Private Lunatic Asylums

Cranborne, Halstock, Stockland

and the foundation of the county asylum at Forston, 1774-1860

Sally Morgan

HOBNOB PRESS

First published in the United Kingdom in 2025
by The Hobnob Press,
8 Lock Warehouse, Severn Road, Gloucester GL1 2GA
www.hobnobpress.co.uk

© Sally Morgan 2025

The Author hereby asserts her moral rights to be identified as the Author of the Work.

All rights reserved. No part of this publication may be reproduced, stored in a retrieval system, or transmitted in any form or by any means, electronic, mechanical, photocopying, recording or otherwise, without the prior permission of the publisher and copyright holder.

British Library Cataloguing in Publication Data
A catalogue record for this book is available from the British Library

ISBN   978-1-918403-02-2

Typeset in Minion Pro, 11/14 pt
Typesetting and origination by John Chandler

Contents

PREFACE

THE TERMINOLOGY USED to describe private asylums and their patients underwent many changes during the centuries discussed in this volume. The terms used here are generally those that were in use by medical professionals and administrators in the 18th and 19th centuries.

In cases where attempts have been made to establish the backgrounds of patients in the asylums and to chart their progress through different institutions the Dorset records have been comprehensively searched. Where patients have resided or been committed to institutions in other counties a much smaller set of sources have been searched.

This volume results from a listing project at the Dorset History Centre to provide access to those records of private asylums retained within the Dorset Quarter Sessions collection. The surviving records include minute books of the visiting officials and inspectors, plans of each asylum, correspondence and case papers. They are a small fraction of the administrative records relating to the asylums. No records of the private asylums are known to survive in private collections. Stories of individual patients were researched within the Herrison Hospital archive which is also held at Dorset History Centre.

ACKNOWLEDGEMENTS

I WOULD LIKE to thank Dr Martin Ayres for supplying references from his research on the Corfe Castle parish collection. Dr Mark Forrest for reading the text and his constant support. Dr John Chandler for typesetting the text and suggested improvements. The earl of Shaftesbury for access to the family and estate archive at Wimborne St Giles. The British Library, The National Archives and Sam Johnston, Dorset County Archivist, for permission to reproduce images. The front of house team at the Dorset History Centre.

Abbreviations

DHC	Dorset History Centre
DvnHC	Devon Heritage Centre
SHC	Somerset Heritage Centre
TNA	The National Archives
WSHC	Wiltshire and Swindon History Centre

'Perhaps any of us, given sufficient provocation, is capable of re-enacting the whole history of the mental health services in personal attitudes – right back to the days of the witch hunts'.
KATHLEEN JONES.[1]

1   Parry-Jones, *English Private Madhouses.*

INTRODUCTION

ASYLUMS IN DORSET AND THE SOUTH-WEST

C ARE FOR INDIVIDUALS suffering from lunacy, madness or mental illness came to the attention of Parliament and the public at large during the reign of George III; perhaps encouraged by the King's own situation. Previously the Court of Wards had managed the affairs of 'idiots' (those unable to care for themselves from birth) and the Court of Chancery oversaw the interests of 'lunatics' (those who had succumbed to, possibly temporary, insanity). Judgements were made by these courts for a small number of wealthy individuals. In most cases family members looked after the patient. When they were unable or unwilling to do so the responsibility fell on the parish to pay for care. This 'care' was provided through a network of houses of private individuals, almshouses, workhouses and private asylums. Inevitably many violent or unruly patients were imprisoned.

In Dorset three private licenced asylums operated during the later part of the 18th century and the first half of the 19th century. At the time these institutions were often referred to as 'madhouses'; reflecting the title of the recently passed 'Act for regulating Private Madhouses' (14 Geo III c.9).[1] The earliest licenced 'house for the reception of *lunaticks*', was established in the parish of Halstock and licenced by the Dorset Quarter Sessions in 1774. A second private asylum in Stockland parish followed and received its 'Madhouse Licence' in 1820.[2] By the time the proprietor of an institution in Cranborne parish applied for its licence in 1830 it was referred to as a 'house for the reception of insane persons'.[3] All three houses were subject to oversight by the Dorset Quarter Sessions which maintained some records of the buildings, administration, proprietors and patients.

---

1   DHC, Q/S/M/1/10, f.100. *Act for Regulating Private Madhouses*, 14 Geo III c.9.

2   DHC, Q/S/M/1/15, f.42.

3   DHC, Q/S/M/1/16, f.156.

Dorset was not unique in hosting a small group of private asylums. During the 18th century a number of small hospitals which fulfilled the role of mental institutions opened in major cities and outside of these areas private asylums were gradually being established.[4] The Country Register, 1798-1812, showed the number of provincial licenced asylums in England (outside the London metropolitan area) in 1802 to be 22, a number which rose to 90 by 1841.[5] These were certainly under estimates which missed some facilities as the existence of the asylum at Halstock, licenced in 1774, was not recognised in the register, such was the unreliable nature of records gathered at the time. An attempt was made to create a comprehensive national list which was published in a Statistical Appendix to the 1844 report of the Metropolitan Commissioners in Lunacy. This included those asylums in the Country Register as well as those in London and others that had not previously been recognised.[6] The dates provided for some of the institutions in the Statistical Appendix related to the commencement date of the surviving records or when the current or previous proprietor took over the establishment. For example the proprietor at Halstock, replied that he had succeeded his aunt, Miss B. Mercer in April 1839, 'and my late mother', however the institution is known to have been in operation from at least 1774. By 1848 the total number of licensed, private, provincial and metropolitan asylums recorded in England and Wales had reached 145.[7]

In 1844 a report of the Metropolitan Commissioners in Lunacy was presented to Parliament by Lord Ashley Cooper who, in 1851, became the 7th Earl of Shaftesbury.[8] The report recognised that Dorset, standing alone amongst counties in the south-west, had established a county asylum which was supported by the county rates under the County Asylums Act of 1808 and the County Asylums Act of 1828.[9] Under the terms of these Acts a county asylum had been opened at Forston in Charminster, near Dorchester, in 1832. For almost two decades the private and county asylums ran in parallel. Until the later 19th century neither the private nor the county asylums had the capacity to manage the number of pauper patients in Dorset and the families of non-pauper patients usually opted to place them in private

4   Rogers, *In the Course of Time*, p.12.

5   Parry-Jones, *The Trade in Lunacy*, pp.30-1.

6   Ibid., p.37.

7   Parry-Jones, *English Private Madhouses*, p.660.

8   *Report of the Metropolitan Commissioners in Lunacy*, 1844.

9   County Asylums Act, 1808, 43 Geo. III, c.96 and County Asylums Act, 1828, 9 Geo. IV, c.40.

houses. Although it had insufficient capacity for all referrals the opening of Forston asylum in 1832 led to the fall in the numbers of pauper patients in Dorset's private asylums.

At Halstock patient numbers peaked in 1825 at 27 of whom nine were paupers. However, between 1830 and 1837 the numbers fell from 23 to just eight who were all private patients. Numbers recovered to the low teens through the next decade though by this time patient classification into pauper and private categories was no longer recorded. Stockland's highest number was recorded in 1830 when it also had a peak of 27 patients. Here the majority, 20, were paupers. Stockland may well have held higher numbers at an earlier date, but records are missing for the previous six years (1824 -1829). In Cranborne the asylum held a maximum of eight private patients in the year 1844.

In 1841, when records are available for all three asylums, there were five private patients at Cranborne, ten private and five pauper patients at Halstock and 14 pauper and 10 private patients at Stockland. General trends across the country show a rise in pauper patients resident in provincial licenced houses outnumbering private patients between 1844 and 1853.[10] However, the picture for this period differs for Dorset, its pauper numbers at the remaining private asylum in Halstock were just two out of 15 patients in 1843.[11] Stockland's asylum had ceased trading by this time and Cranborne continued to receive private patients only. Nationally patient numbers rose in provincial asylums, from 1,321 in 1825 to 3,929 by 1841.[12] Dorset's asylum figures demonstrate an earlier peak in patient numbers, such as at Halstock in 1825; the county generally bucked the national trend for expansion in the 1830s.

Elsewhere in the south-west there were just two county asylums. St Peter's hospital, Bristol was declared a county asylum by a special act of Parliament and a county asylum in Cornwall was supported by a combination of poor rates and public subscriptions; all other institutions in Devon, Somerset and Wiltshire were privately owned and managed until at least 1844.

In the 18th and early 19th centuries pauper lunatics from Dorset parishes were also sent to asylums and hospitals outside the county.[13] Some were committed to London hospitals St Luke's and Bethlem and the asylums at Hindon and Laverstock in Wiltshire and Hoxton, Middlesex. Church

10 Parry-Jones, *The Trade in Lunacy*, p.54.

11 DHC, Q/A/L/Private/1.

12 Parry-Jones, *The Trade in Lunacy*, p.53.

13 Brown, *History of Dorset Hospitals*, p.150.

To have a proper *Petition and Certificate in Order to get* Patients *into* Bethlem-Hofpital.— *It is neceffary to know the following Particulars.*

I. **T**HE Patient's Name and Age—whether married, and how many Children— and what He or She did for a Livelihood, when fenfible ?

II. How long diftracted, and whether ever fo before—and if ftrong enough to take Phyfick ?

III. Whether Melancholy or Raving, and has attempted to do any Mifchief?

IV. Place of the Patient's laft legal Settlement—and how many Church-wardens and Overfeers of the Poor there are in the Parifh ?

V. Some of the Parifh Officers, or fome Relation or Friend of the Patient, is to pe- tition on His or Her Behalf.

N. B. A *Mope*, or one troubled with *Fits*, is *not* a proper Object of the Charity.

The above Particulars being anfwered, a Petition will be drawn at the Clerk's Of- fice, at *Bridewell* Hofpital *(to be Signed by a Governor)* and the Form of a *Certificate*, which is *to be Signed and Sealed* by the Churchwardens and Overfeers of the Poor (of the Parifh where the Patient's Settlement is) in the Prefence of *two Witneffes*, One of whom muft make Oath of the due Execution thereof, before two Juftices of the Peace for the County, or Place, who are to allow the fame, under their Hands.

When the Petition and Certificate are returned, they will be laid before the Com- mittee at *Bethlem* Hofpital, who (fit there *only* on *Saturday* Mornings, from Ten to Eleven o'Clock and) will make an Order as foon as there is a Vacancy, for the Patient to be brought to be Viewed and Examined by them and the Phyfician, and to be then admitted, if a proper Object, that is poor and Mad.

But the Patient muft not be brought up, till fuch an Order is made—and *three Days* before the Time appointed for the Examination, there muft be left at the Clerk's Office, a Note of the Names of two Houfekeepers in *London*, or the Suburbs, who will be prefent at *Bethlem Hofpital at Ten o'Clock in the Morning*, when the Patient is to be admitted, and enter into a Bond of 100 £. to pay for Bedding and Cloaths, during the Patient's Continuance in the Hofpital, and to take Him or Her away when difcharged by the Committee, and to pay the Charge of Burial, if the Patient dies in the Hofpital—And fome Perfon fhould come with the Patient, who can give an Account of the Cafe.

N. B. *No Governor of the Hofpital can be Security for any Patient.*

The process of committal to Bethlem (Bedlam) Hospital (asylum) in Southwark, London, for the year 1768. Those who were 'A Mope' or 'troubled with Fits' were not a 'proper Object of the Charity'. Admittance was only sanctioned after an examination by Bethlem's own physician. It is annotated with a note from Thomas Dawes to his brother William Dawes outlining the required fees. Corscombe parish collection, DHC, PE-COR/OV/10/1.

records held at Dorset History Centre showed Beaminster parish accounts for a pauper lunatic kept at Hindon asylum from April to September 1799 costing £17 including fees for the journey. No indication was given as to why these individuals were confined in asylums outside the county, nor within for that matter, but very likely such asylums were for those who presented challenging behaviours. Whilst it was probably true that the asylum conditions were an improvement on the workhouse; it was certainly a more expensive undertaking for the parish. Similarly, pauper lunatics were placed in the Halstock asylum at some distance from their home these included Ann Davis from Huntsham, Devon, admitted in 1786; Mary Hodder of Plympton, Devon, 1782; James Ross of Holwell, Somerset, 1791; and James Hawkins from Middlezoy, Somerset, 1802.

Contemporary licenced private asylums established in neighbouring counties at the time that Halstock received its first licence in 1774, were few. Wiltshire had the earliest and largest certified institutions in the south-west as well as having more than other counties. The Wiltshire asylums found a role in accommodating the mentally ill outside of London and from adjacent counties. The two notable establishments were Laverstock House and later Fisherton Asylum, both run by the members of the Finch family and situated close to Salisbury.[14] The other early asylums in Wiltshire were Kingsdown House in Box, which may have operated from the early 17th century and Fonthill Gifford which opened in 1718.[15] Laverstock was thought to be operating from the mid 18th century with a great number of pauper lunatics being placed there from outside the county, many were females from the Isle of Wight workhouses.[16] At its height in 1841, it held 135 patients though there was capacity for 50 paupers and 100 private patients. Laverstock's pauper patients were removed to the county asylum at Devizes in 1851, leaving behind 83 private patients.

Fisherton asylum was established in 1813 and it received a large number of patients from east Dorset and Poole where there were no private asylums for either private or pauper patients.[17] Approximately 50 people were registered at Fisherton giving their home parish as Poole between 1813 and 1860 and many more were admitted from the surrounding area. The records of the Guardians of the Poor for the newly formed Poole Poor Law Union provide the opportunity to trace some of these patients over several

14   Newman, 'Laverstock House Asylum', p.105.

15   Parry-Jones, *The Trade in Lunacy*, p.38.

16   Newman, 'Laverstock House Asylum', p.114.

17   WSHC, A1/560/3.

years and sometimes through several different institutions. Ann Moore and David Jacobs who were both sent to Fisherton in October 1836, presumably instead of the workhouse, though no reason was specified.[18] Ann Moore died there after ten years in 1846. David Jacobs was 'relieved' and discharged 14 March 1853, but found admitted to the private asylum at Grove Place in Hampshire, managed by the former proprietor of Cranborne, on 26 March 1853. A year later on 4 May 1854 he was discharged, relieved, only to be found admitted to Hampshire County Asylum on the same day. He was discharged again some years later in February 1862 'not improved'.

Further evidence of patients from the east of the county being cared for at Fisherton asylum can be found in the Corfe Castle overseers records. The document, of 1831, noted that the parish had been supporting two lunatics since 1826 and 1828.[19] It is noted in two letters that one of these lunatics, James Kitcatt, appears to have been confined in Ringwood (Hampshire) asylum in 1811 at a cost of 13s. per week; both letters were signed by C. [Charles] Finch, manager at Fisherton asylum.[20]

The Fisherton and Laverstock asylums were thought to be 'progressive and well run'. Comparisons with other asylums would inevitably be drawn across the county borders, information shared perhaps, particularly when the Commissioners began to undertake visitations of multiple institutions over a wide area, which became standard practice from 1842.

Table 1. The number of private licenced asylums in Dorset and neighbouring counties recorded by the select committees, Parliamentary returns and Metropolitan Commissioners in Lunacy (figures in brackets refer to those receiving paupers).[21]

County	1807	1815	1819	1825	1831	1837	1844	1854
Dorset	1	1	1	2	3	2	2	1
Devon	0	0	0	0	1	3	3 (2)	2 (1)
Hampshire	0	2	2	2	3	5	5 (4)	2 (2)
Somerset	0	1	3	3	4	3	4 (2)	5 (1)
Wiltshire	3	3	5	6	5	7	7 (6)	6 (3)
Total	4	7	11	13	16	20	21 (14)	16 (7)

18 DHC, BG/PL/A/1/1.

19 DHC, PE-COC/OV/11/17. I am indebted to Dr Martin Ayres for supplying this and the following reference.

20 DHC, PE-COC/OV/10/1.

21 Parry-Jones, *The Trade in Lunacy*, pp. 34-5.

During the 19th century the numbers of private licenced asylums were recorded by select committees and parliamentary commissioners. For Dorset their numbers were correct from 1807 until 1831 when all three were recognised as licenced houses. However, three, not two were still operating in 1837. Stockland and Halstock both accommodated paupers throughout their histories until they closed in 1842 and 1858.

Table 2. Statistics from Appendix F of the 1844 report of the Metropolitan Commissioners in Lunacy showing the numbers of pauper lunatics maintained in different classes of accommodation in England and Wales in 1843. Extracted to show provision for Dorset and neighbouring counties.[22]

County	Number of pauper lunatics in county	Number for whom licenced accommodation was available:		Number without licenced accommodation:	
		County asylums; public asylums and hospitals	Private licensed houses	Work-houses	Friends, family or other provision
Dorset	227	97	21	48	44
Devon	547	25	102	145	275
Hampshire	452	3	199	135	115
Somerset	584	12	160	153	259
Wiltshire	373	12	174	73	114
Total	2183	149	656	554	807

Pauper lunatics were housed in different circumstances in the south-west depending upon the provision available. In Dorset, where the county asylum had been established since 1832, it was responsible for a larger share of pauper patients than any other sector. In Wiltshire and Hampshire there were large private asylums and in Somerset and Devon, where there were few comparable institutions, workhouses and private provision made up the great majority of the accommodation.

Dorset's population in the 1841 census was 167,874 of whom 210 people (one in 800) were described in the 1843 abstract of returns, and published in the report of 1844 by the Metropolitan Commissioners in Lunacy, as either a lunatic or an idiot.[23] The returns recorded 127 lunatics (49 male, 78 female) and 83 idiots from birth (33 male and 50 female) within

22   *Report of the Metropolitan Commissioners in Lunacy*, 1844, Appendix F, p.274.
23   Ibid., p.274.

the county; all chargeable to the parishes comprised in each union.

The county lunatic asylum at Forston provided accommodation for 97 (43 male and 54 female), 21 were in in licenced houses (8 male and 13 female), 48 in workhouses (12 male and 36 female) and 44 with friends or elsewhere (19 male and 25 female); the information gathered did not distinguish between lunatics and idiots. The highest number of 50 was expressed for the age group between 40 and 50 years old, followed closely by those 50 to 60 years of age. Further details showed that of these 210 people, 54 were considered to be dangerous to themselves or others and 26 were classed as having 'dirty habits'.

The average weekly cost of maintaining and clothing each individual was also recorded and varied accordingly: Forston county lunatic asylum 7s. 0d., private licenced house 7s. 1½d. and workhouse or family, 2s. 5½d. These official figures seem relatively low and at odds with those recorded in Dorset; Halstock's licenced asylum was charging a basic weekly fee of 12s. some 20 years earlier.

Some understanding of the level of relief Dorset parishes were paying to their poor can be seen in the overseers accounts for Kimmeridge. Although a number of years earlier than the 1844 report, the account for the year 1814 to 1815 shows the parish paid £1 10s., in July 1814, to George Elmes to look after Betty Durham 'when in a deranged state'.[24] In addition Betty received, in 1815, parish relief at 3s. per week which across 50 weeks amounted to £7 10s. This was less than half the cost to Kimmeridge parish of maintaining the criminal lunatic Joseph Whitrow at Halstock.[25] An official return, produced in 1821, indicated that none of its inhabitants were in a workhouse; it seems all were cared for in some way within the parish.

As the provision of county asylum accommodation for paupers expanded, the need for places at the private asylums reduced. This is evident from Halstock's annual register taken in the summer of 1845, where just two patients were paupers out of a total of 16 residents. Cranborne asylum, exclusively for private patients, was caring for six in 1844.[26] The asylum at Stockland had closed in 1842.

The Dorset county asylum at Forston opened in 1832 and by 1842 there was accommodation for 51 male and 62 female paupers. The actual numbers present were 109 by 1842 and 105 by 1843.[27] The county asylum

24 DHC, D-689/1

25 See 'Case Studies', Joseph Whitrow, below.

26 *Report of the Metropolitan Commissioners in Lunacy, 1844*, p.212.

27 Ibid., pp.97 and 132.

provided accommodation for half of those for whom it was required.[28] The remainder were managed in workhouses, as single patients in private houses or sent to institutions in other counties. There was a significant financial incentive to keep paupers within the parish with friends, family, as lodgers or to admit them to the workhouse where the cost was around one third of that charged by a licenced house.

RECORDS OF THE ASYLUMS

UNTIL 1774 THERE was no national scheme for oversight of asylums and consequently very little official record keeping. When lunatics appeared in official records it was usually because a payment was required from their parish or poor law union for maintenance. Legal records were created when disruptive lunatics were brought before the courts, when a guardian was appointed to manage their property or when their assets had been exploited. Probate records might record testamentary bequests to provide long term support. Overall the records are patchy and heavily slanted towards patients who were either particularly dangerous, very wealthy or who required parochial support.

In 1828 the County Asylums Act required that local magistrates sent annual records of admissions, discharges and deaths in asylums to the Home Office, made provision for Justices of the Peace to visit asylums and required that all asylums be certified as suitable for their purpose. Private asylums were regulated and inspected by Visitors appointed at the Quarter Sessions. Their reports, notes, summaries, correspondence and the reactions of the asylum proprietors to them were retained by the court clerk. The Dorset Quarter Sessions collection, relating to the court records for private asylums, and the Herrison hospital collection, relating to both Forston asylum and its successor at Herrison, are held at Dorset History Centre. Although the information regarding patient numbers and details concerning admittance and discharge is patchy and often unreliable there is much to absorb.[29]

The official records are complimented by parish accounts, census returns and court records which supply further detail about the patients, the owners, and the buildings they occupied. Records created at the individual asylums are not known to have survived with the exception of some of the proprietors' correspondence submitted to the Quarter Sessions. No

28 Ibid., pp.84 and 236.
29 DHC, Q/A/L/Private/1-3.

inspections took place of the lodgings where single patients were managed within the parishes and this group remained largely invisible.

The terminology used throughout the Quarter Session court record varied across the decades and changes were made to reflect new thinking and approaches. For consistency and ease of understanding this text uses the terms 'proprietor', 'insane', 'patient' and 'asylum', unless the text is from a direct quote. The Visitors appointed by the Quarter Sessions to inspect the asylums included Justices of the Peace, clergymen, men with some medical background (usually described as surgeons) and members of the local gentry or aristocracy. Collectively they are referred to throughout as the Visitors.

THE PROPRIETORS

IN THE 18TH century asylums in Dorset and other counties were often established by men with some medical training; usually as surgeons. It was also relatively common for those in the medical profession to supplement their income by taking in and supervising a single person with a mental illness within their own homes. This continued without the necessity of a licence until 1829 when the Lunacy Commission were to be informed of the name of any mentally ill patient under the care of a medical man. This list was to remain confidential.[30]

During the late 18th and 19th centuries surgeons were in the middle of the medical hierachy with physicians at the top and the apothecaries at the bottom. Surgeons and apothecaries learned through apprenticeships from masters, and consequently those engaged either of these occupations were considered to be tradesmen rather than professionals. The apothecaries played an important role at grass roots level and by the mid-18th century had assumed the role of a general practitioner. They were more accessible to the general population, particularly the country poor and lower middle classes, and were able to offer medical advice and medicines prepared from plants and minerals. The following description was written by a pamphleteer 1773:

'...Apothecaries have got physic principally into their own hands: this is evidently the case, especially in the country, where the Physician seldom visits any but such as are in opulent circumstances; the poor, alas, scarce

---

30   Brown, *History of Dorset Hospitals*, p.157.

ever! It is much the same in London (allowance being made for those that are in hospitals); so that Apothecaries have by far the greatest number of patients under their own care.[31]

The salaries of those involved in residential medical care was naturally varied. The Dorset example of J. B. Edwards, a surgeon working for the overseers of the poor in Puddletown parish, provides a useful indication his sources of income. Edwards was given a basic retainer of £15 15s., for the year 1812 to 1813, excluding midwifery and surgery.[32] This figure could be expected to more than double for treating the higher society classes on occasion, but generally surgeons and medical men were not considered to be wealthy (compared to their physician counterparts) and this appears to have applied to the three Dorset asylum proprietors. In all three facilities the principal income of the proprietor was derived from the asylum. But, they all found it necessary to engage in other work to supplement their incomes. This involved offering medical services to families in their neighbourhoods, including both the general working population and the local gentry. In Halstock the Mercer family also acted as local apothecaries dispensing drugs, cures and treatments for various ailments. The proprietors at Stockland and Cranborne were engaged in farming.

The three Dorset asylums at Cranborne, Halstock and Stockland were established by surgeons. Occasional references in the Quarter Sessions reports or the census records, indicate that they all lived at their asylums. This may have been viewed as a benefit by the local community as it gave confidence regarding security. The Dorset asylums demonstrated something of a contrast with establishments in other counties where the proprietors often lived elsewhere employing servants to be in charge on site.[33] However, when a resident proprietor was found to be away from the property during times of official visits, their absence was criticised in the Visitors reports.

The proprietors or 'Keepers' of the asylums mentioned in the Dorset Quarter Sessions were, over the years, almost all surgeons, which covered a multitude of medical accomplishments learnt during their apprenticeships. Any experience of the treatment of patients with mental health conditions was acquired during their apprenticeships or through their employment. When an asylum was held by the inheritance of a family member who had

31 Holloway, *The Apothecaries' Act, 1815*, p.1.
32 DHC, PE-PUD/OV/1/51/1.
33 Parry-Jones, *The Trade in Lunacy*, p.89.

not completed an apprenticeship they were obliged to contract in the services of a local surgeon in order to maintain their licence. The apprenticeship of surgeons was overseen by the Company of Barber-Surgeons until 1745, and then by the breakaway Company of Surgeons. Much of their formal training involved surgical procedures and bone fractures, with some dispensary and treatment of common ailments. As training was through apprenticeship, surgeons were likely to develop the specialisms of their masters, and may not have included much mental health care.

In 1800 a royal charter was granted which brought their new title the Royal College of Surgeons of London which, in 1843, was to widen its remit to become the Royal College of Surgeons of England. This led to the insistence from the Royal College of Physicians that to be considered as a member of the Royal College of Surgeons candidates must hold a medical degree. Some visiting medical attendants to the asylums had acquired the M.D. (Doctor of Medicine) qualification which usually meant they had studied in London. Almost all were physicians, university taught, who could diagnose illnesses and prescribe drugs.

THE PATIENTS

I N THE 18TH century legal attitudes towards lunacy were based upon the work of the jurist and legal commentator William Blackstone. In his first volume relating to the laws of England, 'The Rights of Persons', Blackstone discussed the rights in common law regarding 'the custody of idiots, from whence we shall be naturally led to consider also the custody of lunatics'.[34] He continued to describe the distinction between idiots and lunatics: 'An idiot, or natural fool, is one that has had no understanding from his nativity; and therefore is by law presumed never likely to attain any'. A lunatic, or someone described in legal terms as *non compos mentis*, was said to have had understanding

> but by disease, grief, or other accident has lost the use of his reason. A lunatic is indeed properly one that has lucid intervals; sometimes enjoying his senses, and sometimes not, and that frequently depending upon the change of the moon ... in short, as are by any means rendered incapable of conducting their own affairs.

34   Blackstone, *Commentaries on the Laws of England*, vol. I, pp.293-4.

For the legal and medical professions the idiot was thought to be incurable and the lunatic, with supposed temporary mental problems, was expected to make some sort of recovery.

For most people the following generalisation made by Leonard Shelford in 1847 probably reflected the attitudes of the time:

> In common parlance, it is true, some say a person is mad when he does any strange or absurd act; others do not conceive the term madness to be properly applied, unless the person is frantic.[35]

A distinction was made between those people who were a danger to themselves and others, and those who were generally agreeable. The Poor Law Act of 1834 required the removal of dangerous lunatics from public institutions, but because of the additional expense of placing them in the asylum; the large majority of the 'insane' or those with mental health issues remained in the workhouse or as single patients in private houses.

Treatment over the centuries had taken many forms from visits to holy shrines to receiving various apothecary concoctions. The contrasting methods of treatment were highlighted when the Quaker asylum in York, known as the Retreat, which encompassed principles of care and comfort, was established following the death of a Quaker at the York Asylum where the patients were said to be treated worse than animals.[36] The mentally ill poor were the least fortunate, some relied on their families or on charity, some wandered alone in the countryside as was the case for Martha German in 1830, who was found in Devon and subsequently taken to the asylum at Stockland. Those likely to harm others or themselves would result in time spent in the stocks, chained up or imprisoned.[37]

The Earl of Shaftesbury, involved with the subject of lunacy from 1829, provided detailed comments alongside parliamentary minutes of evidence dated 1859. Within this document he defined people who were thought of and described as 'dangerous' - he said the formula often used was *'None but those who are dangerous to themselves or others'*. He went on to say that there was *'no notion'* of what people in society meant by the word dangerous and qualified his thoughts further by stating it was:

---

35 Shelford, *Definition of Sound and Unsound Mind*, p.41.

36 Tuke, *Description of the Retreat*.

37 Rogers, *In the Course of Time*, p.12.

not necessary to be suicidal, or homocidal, to be dangerous to himself or others - Idiots, Paralytics, Epileptics, Imbeciles, may fall down stairs, out of the window, into the fire, may be suffocated in bed, are utterly unable to help themselves in any way.

He recognised that some people were 'fearfully noisy' and harassed and terrified neighbourhoods day and night. Difficult enough to manage in a large property 'aided by wealth and solitude', he questioned the ability of carers to cope in 'a very small house - a Shop Keeper's perhaps - with very many small children, and limited means?' His concern was for society as well as to the patient: how family members, neighbours and the broader community might be adversely effected by the lunatic, as well as the treatment and care of the lunatic themselves. Shaftesbury described how a man could ruin his family by wild expenditure and then throw them on the state or on relatives. In his example he said a man with £600,000 could buy a tea-cup for £6,000 without endangering his dependents and perhaps be considered eccentric, but a man with only £6,000, with a family, doing the same could be thought of as being a 'madman'. He suggested that 'such a one, being of unsound mind, is not dangerous?' and that if so everyone of unsound mind should be retained. But, 'No - we must, in consideration of the great principle of Liberty, be prepared to incur many hazards.'[38]

Those who could not be looked after at home had few choices, largely governed by the ability of their family to pay for care or treatment. Some were able to live at home, buying in care, whilst others were lodged with families who supplemented their income by providing this service for one or two residents. No certification was required by the Quarter Session, these houses were entirely unregulated, and no mandatory checks were made by court or parish officials. However, they might achieve some quasi-official status by receiving residents who were partly supported by poor relief paid by the parish officers. Such houses were often known locally as the 'Madhouse'. Some of these institutions which sprang up to cope with local needs were the origins of the madhouses for the private lunatics. Too expensive for many, and unavailable in many parishes, the pauper lunatics were more likely to be granted space in an almshouse or a workhouse. Those who were challenging in their behaviour or thought to be dangerous were put into a separate building close or adjacent to the workhouse known as the blind house; usually intended for people who misbehaved.[39]

38   Shaftesbury estate archive, SE/P/39.

39   Brown, *History of Dorset Hospitals*, p.149.

Many mentally ill people, whether they were privately funded or paupers, often had their admission to private asylums delayed despite the known value of early intervention or treatment.[40]For paupers this was mainly ascribed to miserly tendencies on the part of parish officials. For the privately funded, this was attributed to the 'ignorance, wickedness or desire for secrecy of relatives', financial issues and property holdings probably played their part too. The outcome in both cases was that people were generally only placed into an asylum when their condition became unmanageable and 'physically dilapidated' which resulted in any improvement, or cure even, virtually impossible.

Lord Malmesbury commented on this situation in the second reading of what became the Lunatic Asylums Act of 1828 that the intention and object of the bill was to enable magistrates to increase the allowances given by parishes to private houses. He further said that one of the *'greatest evils'* of the previous system was that a parish would seek an asylum for a pauper lunatic which was the cheapest. Inevitably asylum keepers were in competition which resulted in accepting an allowance of 9s. per week. This amount could only provide basic food and lodging, certainly no curative treatment which, if it had, a recovery might have been possible. He continued:

> It consequently happened, that individuals sent to those asylums, who might have recovered had medical treatment been given to them, remained in them beyond the time when recovery might be hoped for, and became incurable lunatics. That evil would be got rid of by the present bill; for its object was to provide asylums, not only for the reception, but for the cure of insane persons.[41]

In 1836, an Assistant Poor Law Commissioner succinctly summed up the situation for paupers in his county of Devon:

> At the moment we do not know what to do with a pauper lunatic . . . I believe that many lunatic paupers might have been cured if the disorder had been properly treated at an early stage, but the expense of sending them to an asylum, there being no county asylum, is so great, that they have been kept in the workhouses until they become so troublesome, that it is desirable to remove them even at considerable expense; but in the meantime the disease has become inveterate and recovery is hopeless.

40   Parry-Jones, *The Trade in Lunacy,* pp.247-9.

41   Hansard, *Lunatic Asylums Regulation Bill,* (HL Deb 29 April 1828 v. 29 cc196-97).

The rise of pauper numbers can be attributed to economic changes generated by the Industrial Revolution and rapid population increase.[42] Rural farming communities were deeply affected resulting in increased poverty, the distress of which often led to the downward spiral of mental illness in its many forms. As greater attention was paid, more cases of insanity were reported. Official figures gathered in 1844, suggested the number of pauper and private patients considered insane across England and Wales and residing in asylums and other institutions, to be almost 21,000.

With regard to the Dorset private asylums the situation relating to pauper and private patients is opaque. Cranborne received no pauper patients. Halstock was certainly taking pauper patients from its establishment in 1775, but no record was made of how their admission and treatment differed from that of the private patients, if it differed at all. In many of the Halstock and Stockland returns and reports it is impossible to distinguish between pauper and private patients. For those where the distinction can be made, it appears that Stockland housed more pauper lunatics than Halstock. At a cost of anything between 8s. and 14s. per week the private asylum was an expensive undertaking for a parish, domestic care or the workhouse being the cheaper options. Those people who found themselves confined as a lunatic generally fared better in the private asylum than in the workhouse or private house as there was, to some limited extent, an attempt made towards treatment and rehabilitation.[43] Perhaps some of those who were afforded a more immediate entry into a private asylum benefitted from a local benefactor or perhaps families contributed somehow, in some small way.[44]

Reasons for confinement and the character of the patient were rarely given in any of the Dorset asylums, perhaps because they were of little interest to the court of Quarter Sessions. Private or pauper, there were no references to people with obvious physical disabilities, nor were any difficulties presented in relation to placing pauper lunatics into private asylums alongside private patients, but presumably accommodation and staffing played a part especially for those considered dangerous. Occasionally references were made during official visits which described patients as 'dangerous' as was the case regarding Edward Lloyd, a private patient at Cranborne.

42   Parry-Jones, *The Trade in Lunacy*, p.13.

43   Brown, *History of Dorset Hospitals*, p.151.

44   See below for the case of Elizabeth Nation, a patient at Cranborne admitted at the age of 13.

For the parish officers determining how best to deal with members of their community there were choices to be made, both relating to the care of the patient and the parish finances. Table 3 displays a return 'of all Lunatics and dangerous Idiots' made by the overseers of the poor of Broadwindsor, in west Dorset, in 1838/9.[45] This took place six years after the founding of the county asylum and the suggestion in the Poor Law Amendment Act that (dangerous) lunatics should not be kept in the workhouse for more than 14 days. At Broadwindsor the overseers confirmed that only one had been admitted to Forston, three remained in the workhouse and two were at liberty within the parish receiving unspecified support.

Table 3. Return of the overseers of the poor of Broadwindsor in 1838/9.

1838	Age	Whether Lunatic or Idiot	Whether dangerous or otherwise	For what length of time disordered in his or her senses	Where confined, and since what time	At what expense
Samuel Randle	58/59	Idiot	not dangerous	From infancy	In workhouse, not confined	
Bridget Crocker	51	Lunatic	not dangerous	18 years	In workhouse, not confined	
William Peters	44	Lunatic	occasionally dangerous	20 or 21 years	Not under confinement at present	
John Symes	25	Idiot	not dangerous	12 or 13 years	Not under confinement	
William Payne	17	Idiot	not dangerous	From infancy	In workhouse	
William Peters	50	Lunatic	occasionally dangerous	24 or 25 years	In County Asylum Forston	6s. 5d. per week
1839						
William Peters	about 53			25 or 26 years		
Samuel Priest	about 46		dangerous (?) about a year ago			

45   DHC, PE-BDW/OV/10/1/1.

Some details of one of the Broadwindsor lunatics can be assembled from which it appears that only those who might be considered dangerous were sent to an asylum. William Peters had been admitted register to Stockland asylum in 1831, when his home parish was given as Broadwindsor. At his confinement in 1831 he was thought to be 'curable' and was released two years later 'cured'. But the following year, in 1834, he was admitted to Forston asylum. His cause of insanity was given as receiving blows to the head, he was said to be violent and disposed to idleness and drinking.[46] He was released and re-admitted in 1836,[47] None of the others listed in 1838 appear in the records of Stockland or Forston asylums. Samuel Priest's admission papers to Forston show that he was admitted in November 1838,[48] and was probably only listed by the Broadwindsor overseers in 1839 when they were required to make their first payment for his care. In the admission papers he was described as violent and with a disposition to destroy his clothes. His condition was considered to be both hereditary and caused by a blow to the head.

The Parliamentary committee which had investigated better asylum regulation in England 1815 discussed, with evidence, the many aspects of care which might influence treatment and recovery. One aspect was one of overcrowding '*Keepers of the houses receiving a much greater number of persons in them than they are calculated for*' and it was noted that this '*retards recovery*'.[49] It was considered that some private asylums were taking in numbers of lunatics above their licence quota. It is possible that proprietors were under pressure to oblige despite the overcrowding, or perhaps it was simple greed. Looking after larger numbers, with few staff, would have undoubtedly led to many patients being held in restraint, an outcome recognised by the same committee and considered unsatisfactory.[50]

ACTS OF PARLIAMENT

PRIVATE ASYLUMS AND madhouses had been present in England as unregulated institutions since at least the end of the 16th century. In 1763 a Parliamentary committee found that many sane people had been

46 DHC, NG-HH/CMR/4/32A/104.

47 DHC, NG-HH/CMR/4/32A/150.

48 DHC, NG-HH/CMR/4/32A/243.

49 *First Report from the Committee on the State of Asylums*, I.

50 Ibid., II, p.5.

placed in these institutions. Some were confined for financial reasons, to exploit their assets, others for social reasons, including to remove an unwanted partner or to conceal an illicit relationship. The need to regulate private asylums resulted in five significant Acts of Parliament introduced during the years in which the Dorset asylums operated: Act for Regulating Private Madhouses, 1774, the County Asylums Act 1808, the Madhouse Act 1828, the Lunacy Act 1842, and the Lunacy Act 1845.

Between 1774 and 1900 a total of 43 Acts of Parliament were passed which focused directly on the care and rights of lunatics in England and Wales (see Appendix 5). Many of these Acts remained on the statute books until they were consolidated and updated in the 1959 Mental Health Act. Additionally numerous Acts relating to workhouses, prisons, parish poor relief (particularly the Poor Law Amendment Act, 1834) and local government contained clauses that that applied to their treatment and accommodation. The principal acts relating to the management of asylums are detailed below.

The Act for Regulating Private Madhouses, 1774.
Whether for private or pauper lunatics, legislation defined the history of the private madhouse system, first by the Private Madhouses Act of 1774.[51] This Act was introduced largely as a result of increasing public concern that non-lunatics were being detained by members of their family for no good reason and stories of abuses and brutal neglect were published in pamphlets and articles.[52] Its primary purpose was aimed at regulating both the private trade in lunacy and the keeping of more than one patient in a private house. The three main provisions were that a limit was to be placed on the number of patients admitted, medical certificates were needed for confinement and admissions notified within 14 days to the Commissioners in Lunacy in London, though in this last matter paupers were excluded. Most importantly this Act determined that asylums could not operate without a licence or regular inspections.

The asylums were to be inspected once a year and, outside of London, this task would be carried out by local Justices of the Peace, made up of some gentry, clerics and members of Parliament. They would also keep a central register of all the confined lunatics. In reality licences were rarely, if ever, refused and inspections were superficial making the resulting reports worthless.

51   Act for Regulating Private Asylums, 1774, 14 Geo. III, c.49.
52   Parry-Jones, *The Trade in Lunacy,* p.9.

The Act required that a record be made of the Justices' visits to the private asylums and in Dorset the earliest licenced house at this time was Halstock. Their task was to place on record general observations and names of those incarcerated, notes were also made on the general state of the patients and their accommodation and reported to the court. Suggestions were made on matters of improvement on rare occasions, treatments were not. The Visitors had virtually no power and the reality of the new regime was little more than a formality, but it was a beginning of sorts to expedite future change.[53] It survived, without amendment for 54 years.

The County Asylums Act 1808

The County Asylums Act of 1808, also known as the Lunatic Paupers or Criminals Act 1808 or Wynn's Act, allowed county administrations to provide asylums, but did not compel them to do so.[54] The intention was to provide appropriate facilities for pauper lunatics who were receiving inadequate care in workhouses and prisons. In anticipation of the Act the Dorset Clerk of the Peace sent a circular to the overseers of the poor in Dorset parishes requesting that an account of all lunatics and insane persons confined within Dorset establishments should be delivered to the clerk in Shaftesbury by 29 March 1806.[55]

The Act provided the blueprint (specifications) for the building and continuing support of what would be publicly funded county asylums, its mission was 'for the better Care and Maintenance of Lunatics, being Paupers or Criminals, in England'. Progress was slow, across the first 20 years only nine counties built asylums, thought due in part to a reluctance to raise the initial funds and concerns about the future costs.[56]

The County Asylums Act and Madhouse Act, 1828.

Eventually, after 54 years, the Act for Regulating Private Madhouses was replaced in 1828 by the County Asylums Act, relating to the erection and regulation of asylums, and the Madhouse Act relating to the care and treatment of insane persons.[57] Annual licences, now to include a plan of the premises, would continue to be sought and granted by the court, but

53 Brown, *History of Dorset Hospitals*, p.158.
54 County Asylums Act, 48 Geo. III, c.96.
55 DHC, PE-WOR/OV/6/1.
56 Jones, *Lunacy, Law and Conscience*, pp.74-5.
57 County Asylum Act, 1828, 9 George IV c.40. The Madhouse Act 1828, 9 George IV c.41.

now with additional legislation which included the overseeing of the management of both private and pauper patients.[58] The officials, Justices of the Peace, could also now refuse to renew a licence[59] Two court officials and a medical visitor, appointed at the local Quarter Sessions, were to visit at least four times a year and submit a report to the Secretary of State.

A more explicit form of certification was required for the purpose of preventing illegal detention, officials now had the power to release those thought to be improperly confined. Admissions were to be notified to the official clerk within seven days and three days where a patient had died or been removed. Asylums with under 100 patients were to have a visit from a doctor to assess the health of the patients and condition of the house once or twice a week. The doctor would report their findings to the proprietor. Divine service was to be made available for all each Sunday and relatives or 'friends', who had originally authorised the patient's admission, were to visit every six months.

Records of the number of curable and incurable male and female patients and their general condition were to be kept by the proprietor along with information of those under restraint. Additionally, if malpractice was suspected, visits could be made, both announced and unannounced, during the night.

The Visitors who were appointed under the terms of the Acts were to ensure that such malpractice did not take place. Halstock was visited by two or three Justices of the Peace, a physician and clerk three times in the first year of the Madhouse Act, and continued to have regular visits, averaging four times a year, until 1842. Stockland, as recorded by the court, received fewer, on average three visits per year. Cranborne was also inspected regularly, usually three times each year, though there were some years missed. There is no suggestion that night visits were ever made at any of the Dorset asylums.

Records were to be kept which included a book in which the court officials were to report the condition of the house, report on the care of the patients and note when religious aid (divine service) was offered. Under the terms of the Madhouse Act it became necessary to advise the Justices of all admissions. Justices of the Peace for the first time acquired the power to refuse a licence. The Visitors also had the power to release anyone thought to have been improperly confined following three visits with 21 days between each visit.

58   Jones, *Lunacy, Law and Conscience,* p.143.
59   Brown, *History of Dorset Hospitals,* p.160.

The Poor Law Act of 1834.
The Poor Law amendment act of 1834 stated that 'nothing in this Act contained shall authorise the detention in any workhouse of any dangerous lunatic, insane person, or idiot for any longer period than fourteen days'. The Metropolitan Commissioners chose to interpret this as prohibiting the detention of all lunatics, whereas the Poor Law Commissioners interpreted it as applying only to dangerous lunatics. Under either interpretation this was the first time that restrictions had been imposed on the length of time that a lunatic, idiot or insane person could be maintained in a workhouse.

The Lunacy Act, 1842
Though not as new or wide ranging as some of the earlier Acts, or the Act that replaced it three years later, the Lunacy Act 1842 marked a significant regulatory change.[60]The Earl of Shaftesbury, already a national figure, was the acknowledged leader of lunacy reform and, together with other like minded peers, he sought to cease the unsatisfactory situation of divided authorities and responsibilities.[61]

The powers of the Metropolitan Commissioners were extended to include the provinces.[62]They were directed to visit and inspect all the public and private asylums throughout England and Wales, excepting Bethlem. Their subsequent report made to the Lord Chancellor in 1844 contained the first comprehensive survey of provincial private licenced houses. Many recommendations made in this report were later embodied in the Lunatics Act of 1845. Years later, in 1882, D H Tuke referred to the report as 'the Doomsday Book of all that concerns institutions for the insane at that time'.

In practice this meant in addition to the usual visits by local Justices of the Peace, Metropolitan Commissioners in Lunacy, which included a physician and barrister, were required to visit licenced houses outside the London area twice a year. They were to receive five guineas a day.[63] Evidence of fact finding while drafting the Act can be seen in a letter, written in the midst of 1842, to Mr Fooks, clerk of the peace in Sherborne, from the Metropolitan Commissioners in Lunacy in London, requesting information as to the existence of '*any County Lunatic asylum and also what licensed Houses and where situate (sic) within your district*'. Fooks replied that there was a

60   The Lunacy Act, 1842, 5 & 6 Victoria, c.87.

61   Jones, *Lunacy, Law and Conscience*, p.170.

62   Parry-Jones, *The Trade in Lunacy,* p.20

63   Jones, *Lunacy, Law and Conscience*, p.174.

County Lunatic asylum at Forston and two licenced houses, Halstock and Cranborne. Stockland was not mentioned, although it was still operating as an asylum in Dorset at this time; the parish was formally transferred to Devon in 1844.[64]

In addition to these changes the Commissioners were required to report on the continuing practice of mechanical restraint. This had been abolished in June 1841, largely due to the influence of the enlightened Mr Gaskell, under whose influence forms of occupational therapy were beginning to be recognised as beneficial.[65] Gaskell had been appointed medical superintendent at the large county asylum in Lancashire and his ideas had a considerable influence upon the Earl of Shaftesbury.

Lunacy Act and County Asylums Act 1845.
The Lunacy and County Asylums Acts of 1845 had been passed partly to quicken the progress of establishing county asylums.[66] The Lunacy Act related to the inspection of asylums and provision of medical staff, while the County Asylums Act made the provision of an asylum compulsory in every county. The Metropolitan Commissioners were now replaced by the Board of Commissioners in Lunacy whose existence was created to provide a coherent permanent and central supervising body.[67] This new board of Commissioners of eleven was headed by the Earl of Shaftesbury. Six of the commissioners, three medical men and three from the legal profession, received a remuneration of £1,500 per year plus travel expenses; making their roles full-time salaried posts. The remaining five commissioners were unpaid honorary members who attended board meetings only.

Besides Shaftesbury, who was chair until his death in 1885, the honorary members were laymen: Lord Seymour (formerly Lord Granville Somerset), Vernon Smith, Robert Gordon and Francis Barlow. Of these Robert Gordon and Lord Seymour visited Halstock and the Earl of Shaftesbury visited Cranborne, close to his home at Wimborne St Giles. All three medical Commissioners Thomas Turner, Henry Southey and John Hume inspected Halstock and Cranborne. The three legal Commissioners James Mylne, Bryan Proctor and John Hall all visited Halstock and Mylne

---

64 DHC, Q/A/L/Private/1.
65 Jones, *Lunacy, Law and Conscience*, p.174.
66 The Lunatics Act, 1845, 8 & 9 Victoria, c.100. County Asylums Act, 1845, 8 & 9 Victoria, c.126.
67 Parry-Jones, *The Trade in Lunacy*, p.20.

and Proctor both visited Cranborne.[68] Stockland asylum had closed before the Commissioners began their visits.

The newly appointed and named Lunacy Commissioners were to continue with the inspection, licensing and reporting duties of the former Metropolitan Commissioners. Their existing functions remained almost unchanged, and now inspection duties were extended to all licenced asylums and hospitals in the country. Visits were to take place by one medical and one legal Commissioner twice a year in the provinces at any time of day. The Commissioners were to check on those patients under medical restraint, inspect records and report on the outbuildings. They were also able to discharge patients after two visits following an interval of seven days if they considered that they should be released. Reports of all inspections were made to the Lord Chancellor three times a year.[69] Local Justices of the Peace continued to make their visits independent of the Commissioners.

Improvements to certification was made which increased safeguards against wrongful confinement. Asylums were also required to keep six record books: an admissions book, a book for recording discharge, death or transfer to another establishment, a medical casebook, a medical visitation book, a patients' book for observations on individuals and a visitors book.[70] The medical visitation book was for the first time intended to provide a record of treatment, any form of restraint, details of seclusion or irregular confinement, and a record of injuries and violent incidents. The visitors book was to include both official reports and unofficial notes and observations. New attention was to be paid to the diet of pauper patients which was to be regulated if necessary. A provision was also included to allow patients to spend time away from the asylum, with consent, for a short time as a benefit to their health.

The passing of the 1845 Lunacy Act and County Asylums Act was the culmination of years of debate and investigation largely driven by the 7th Earl of Shaftesbury and other like-minded individuals. By involving inspectors from outside the county community and enhancing recording and reporting mechanisms it had a significant impact. It also marked a change in the language first used in 1774, 100 years earlier, from 'Lunatick or mad person' to a 'person of unsound mind'.[71]

68   Jones, *Lunacy, Law and Conscience*, p.191.

69   Ibid., pp.191-2.

70   Ibid., p.194.

71   Ibid., p.195.

THE EFFECTS OF THE ACTS

SOME OF THE Visitors might be considered enlightened, while others remained more traditional in their views. The enlightened view was reflected in the gradual change in the language used to describe those confined from the terms 'idiot' and 'lunatick' to the general use of 'inmate' or 'patient', which became standard by the mid-19th century. However, a lapse into a more traditional mindset can be found as in the December of 1847 when Visitors John Goodden and W. J. Goodden observed at Halstock that the 'Prisoner (was) more than usually dirty but again difficult to keep clean'.

Alongside the changing legislation the plight of the insane was brought to the public through articles published in newspapers. One publication used satire to make its point. In 1839 an article entitled Madhouses and their Management, the 'Satirist; or the Censor of the Times', used this style of humour to comment on the licensed private asylums in England.[72] Representing Dorset, Stockland and Halstock asylums fared well, they were listed together with with their proprietors and patient numbers without further comment. In contrast, Gateshead had four establishments one of which was accommodating twelve more women than men leading to the comment regarding the supposed level of protection given by their male proprietors. A case 'of scandalous misconduct' at York asylum, regarding the birth of a child, bore similarities to the situation which took place at Halstock almost a decade later. Grove Place at Nursling, later to be managed by Cranborne's William Symes, is mentioned because a murder had been committed there; Cranborne asylum itself was not included in the report. Hertfordshire and Kent are castigated for lack of proper returns whilst Hereford passes without comment. Several counties failed to provide any returns.

In 1842, the Commissioners conducted a 'tour of inspection' of the 99 English private asylums outside the jurisdiction of the metropolitan area of London.[73] Rather than discovering extensive cruelty and neglect they found a common theme of law evasion. Confirmation was also made of the generally held view that asylum proprietors frequently took their responsibilities somewhat casually. In this aspect Cranborne's proprietor drew criticism for

---

72 *The Satirist; or, the Censor of the Times*, 14 April 1839.

73 Jones, *Lunacy, Law and Conscience*, p.178.

MADHOUSES AND THEIR MANAGEMENT.

In the disclosure of some of the most flagrant of the abuses that were detected by Mr. Godfrey Higgins, as having been practised in secrecy or in connivance, at the York Asylum, another case of scandalous misconduct is presented, as regards the laxity of discipline in the place, and the gross and criminal indecencies permitted towards the female patients. That persevering gentleman discovered that an inmate of the establishment, named DorothyExilby, of Kirby Malzeard, had been admitted in the month of February, and discharged as cured in the February following. That she had brought a child into the world in the month of September, but there was a difficulty, arising from private reasons, in finding out the father, though it was strongly supposed he was, or rather it was charged upon one of the patients. A similar circumstance occurred in the case of a lady in a superior situation in life, who was placed there for proper treatment under mental disease, and who was let out in a state of infamous disgrace ; but a feeling of delicacy restrained the publicity of further notice of the foul affair, though the author of her misfortune was some person wi h'n the house. Instances of neglect, cruelty, and unnecessary severity in that Asylum, are numerous, some of which shall be exposed.

We have on a former occasion given our readers a very accurate list of the Private Lunatic Asylums within seven miles round London, licensed by the Metropolitan Commissioners in Lunacy, under the provisions of the Act 2d and 3d William IV. We now furnish, as correctly as the returns enable us to prepare it, a list of the licensed Asylums in England and Scotland, with the number of inmates, male and female, in each. We only wish that we could, in addition, at present hand up the names of these inmates, as we are perfectly convinced that publicity alone can effect any reform in the present abominable system, and afford security to personal liberty.

It will be observed that from several of the counties there is no return at all ; and with regard to such returns as have been made, much latitude is to be given for wilful suppression and misrepresentation.

An article published in the Satirist *in April 1839, under the title 'Madhouses and their Management', listed and commented on the licensed private asylums in England. They considered that reform of the 'present abominable system' could only be achieved by publicity which included presenting the names of those confined*

(continued on next page).

his absence on three occasions at the time of Commissioner's visits. Symes was not alone, absences at times of Visits were also recorded at Stockland and Halstock. The findings of the Commissioners' tour resulted in the publication of the report of 1844, compiled and written by Lord Ashley (7th Earl of Shaftesbury).[74]

It had been suspected by the Commissioners that across the country not all local magistrates took their duties under the various Lunacy Acts

74　Ibid., p.175

LICENSED PRIVATE ASYLUMS IN ENGLAND.

DORSET.

Situation.	Proprietor	m	f.
Boardhay's House, Stockland	William Spicer	9	8
Halstock............................	Alice Mercer—Betsy Mercer	17	10

DURHAM.

Gateshead Fell	John Orton......................	22	12
Bencham, Gateshead	Frederick Glenton—Paul Glenton--	22	34
The Flatts, ditto	William Oxley, M. D.............	11	14
Gateshead Fell, ditto	Jacob Gowland .... unknown—suppose 25.		

Note.—Here we have a whole parish devoted to the trade in lunacy, containing on a moderate calculation one hundred and forty patients. There must be a wide field for the investigation of abuses here. What! 34 ladies under the protection of. Messrs. Glenton !!!

ESSEX.

Witham...	Thomas Tomkin.................	8	1
Leopard's-hill Lodge, Loughton....	Matthew Allen M.D.	2	2

(Much underrated.)
Note.—Is the solitary female with Mr. Tomikin likely to recover her proper state of mind without the society of her sex?

GLOUCESTER.

Fishponds, Stapleton...... -.......	George G. Bompass, M.D.	27	24
Ridgeway House, ditto	Nehemiah Duck..................	6	13
Fairford............ -...........	Alexander Iles...................	6	3

HAMPSHIRE.

Grove-place, Nursling ·· ··········	Benjamin Middleton, M.D.........	30	26
Newport, Isle of Wight	William Hearne	10	16

Note.—The house at Grove-place is that where the unfortunate Mrs. Strong was murdered—a case still fresh in the recollection of our readers.

HEREFORD.

Hereford Asylum, Hereford City....	John S. L. Pateshall	15	7
Peterchurch House, Peterchurch ..	Simon Exton, M.D.	3	1

HERTFORDSHIRE.

Little Hadham.....................	Mary Jacob	7	6

Note.—This is a very insufficient return ; there was and no doubt is a house at Hertford and another at Ware.

KENT.

West Malling-place, near Maidstone	Robert Rix	23	14

Note.—Insufficient again ; there is a house at Sevenoaks, and another at Tunbridge Wells, and one near Margate.

(To be continued.)

seriously, with some not visiting the asylums at all. Dorset asylums were generally inspected more regularly than those in other counties, usually receiving their quota of visits, with only a few lapses which might be accounted for by clerical or procedural errors.

Magistrates who were conscientious in their inspections might differ in their personal areas of interest. Stockland Visitors in 1837 were keen to report on details of the patient's diet, but this subject was not mentioned at all at Halstock, and at Cranborne mealtimes were noted but the food was not. At all asylums the focus was placed on cleanliness of the house, the patients and their bedding, often describing the 'wards' as being in a 'wholesome' state.

At all three asylums observations were particularly made whether patients were in an '*excited*' state. This condition continued to be noted across subsequent visits with patients recorded as being in a more or less '*excited*' state (1833-1834). The times when patients were found to be '*tranquil*' were also clearly recorded (1835). This behaviour was not explained though it is possible the term '*excitement*' was used when any witnessed behaviour was not considered to be normal. Sometimes disruptive behaviour, along with excessive energy levels, resulted in a '*degree of coercion*' used in order to keep either the 'excited' individual safe from self-harm or from inflicting harm upon other patients (1837).

All aspects of ventilation featured heavily in reports made to the court; there was always a great importance placed on being able to declare the rooms free of '*offensive smells*'. The Visitors reported very little concerning medical treatment, it was of no statutory importance. Nor were they particularly concerned with the employment of patients in any form of work or activities, it was a subject given only a light touch, with few recommendations.

A BRIEF CHRONOLOGY OF ASYLUMS IN DORSET

THE FIRST RECORDED asylum in Dorset, at Halstock, was already open when it was licenced according to the new law in 1774. Stockland asylum was licenced in 1820 and Cranborne asylum in 1830.

In 1807 there were 110 recorded cases of lunacy among paupers in Dorset who required financial support. The breakdown of these cases shows 47 kept in the workhouse, 41 in private custody (including private asylums) and 22 not confined but maintained by the parish.[75] This figure was published in 1808 as part of a 'Plan for the Division of the Kingdom into Districts, for the Erection of Lunatic Asylums'. Dorset was linked in the plan with the counties of Wiltshire and Hampshire, with a proposed site for an asylum at Salisbury.[76] This plan was never to be realised and was superseded by the provisions for county asylums. But, it demonstrates that the problem had been recognised and that some efforts were already being made to establish what accommodation was required.

Dorset's new public asylum opened at Forston near Charminster in 1832.[77] Neighbouring counties were still some years behind: Devon in

---

75   Brown, *History of Dorset Hospitals*, p.149

76   *Report from the Select Committee on the State of Lunatics*, 1808, p.144.

77   Rogers, *In the Course of Time*, p.14.

1845, then Somerset 1848, Wiltshire 1851 and finally Hampshire in 1852. Many of the paupers from Dorset private asylums, particularly Halstock and Stockland, can be found in the early admission registers and order papers for Forston.[78] Some were then moved to their home county asylums at a later date as the pressure for places grew.

The opening of the county asylum probably accelerated the closing of the three asylums earlier than in other counties. Stockland closed in 1841, Cranborne in 1848 and finally Halstock in 1858. In some counties private asylums continued to handle paupers well into the second half of the 19th century due to delays in building; even taking in patients from those institutions already overcrowded.[79]

78   DHC, NG-HH/CMR/4.

79   Parry-Jones, *English Private Asylums*, p.660.

THE EARLIEST DORSET ASYLUMS.

DORSET ASYLUMS AND PROVISION FOR THE
MENTALLY ILL BEFORE 1774

IT IS HARD to ascertain what provisions were made for the mentally ill in Dorset before 1774. A few scattered references supply details of isolated cases. In 1623 the burgesses of Bridport borough bound Robert Balston to take in his brother Phillip, a lunatic, who had threatened and beaten people in the town and neighbourhood.[80] This was a community response from Bridport and Robert was given an annual allowance of 40s. to care for his brother. In 1758 William Walrond was appointed guardian for the Dorset property of George Larder, a lunatic.[81] In 1772 John Dennett of Blandford Forum left a trust in his will for the Revd Butt to administer on behalf of Mary Muston, a lunatic.[82] The Lyme Regis overseers of the poor paid 3s. 3d. for 'guarding and maintaining Robert Brown, a lunatic, in 1773.[83] These brief references, and others scattered through the accounts of parish churchwardens, relate to the responsibility of providing maintenance or the management of an estate. They provide no information about where these patients were housed, the nature of their illnesses, whether any treatment was offered, their living conditions or who cared for them.

Only at Halstock is it possible to obtain some insight into the lives of the patients beyond the financial responsibility for their care. The first reference to an asylum in the small village of Halstock can be found in a document dated 1722 when Edward Symes was paid for keeping a lunatic, Sarah Norwood, from Lyme Regis.[84] She was described as '*being disordered in her senses*'. It was not unusual at the time for those in the

80   DHC, DC-BTB/M/27.
81   DHC, D-RGB/KF/20.
82   DHC, D1/9661.
83   DHC, PE-LR/OV/1/1.
84   DHC, DC-LR/M/4, p.13.

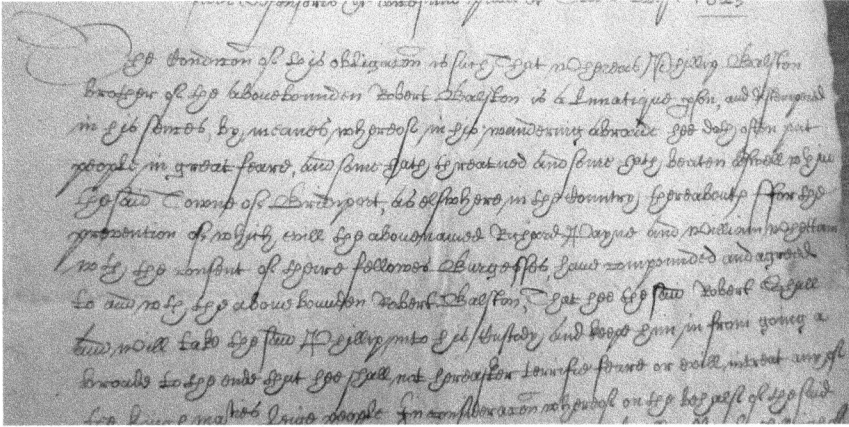

Bond by which the bailiff's of Bridport and Robert Balston arranged the care of Phillip Balston, 1623. DHC, DC-BTB/M/27.

medical profession to provide a 'home' for someone deemed mad. It paid well; Symes received an annual payment of £10 8s. 0d. from the Lyme Regis overseers.

A few years later in his will of 1729 Edward Symes, who was described as a physician, bequeathed £10 to a Thomas Mercer.[85] Thomas was the first of the Mercer dynasty to be recorded caring for lunatics in Halstock. Although there is no evidence of an apprenticeship, it seems likely Thomas Mercer accumulated medical knowledge from Edward Symes which enabled him to continue caring for the insane within the village. Symes himself may have been part of a wider county network of medical men: in 1729 a Robert Symes of the nearby village of Netherbury married Joan the daughter of William Wiseman a physician of Weymouth.[86]

The Quarter Session minutes recorded the first reference to the Mercer family independently providing care for an individual suffering from mental illness. In 1747 Thomas Mercer of Halstock was awarded a court order of £18 for:

> dyet and clothing one Bynen a person committed to his custody by the Order of this Court who was furiously Mad and for his care and medicines used in curing him of his said madness'[87]

85   WSHC, P16/255 (1729).

86   DHC, D1/9732.

87   DHC, Q/S/M/1/8.

The previous year the same person, Peter Bynen, had been ordered in the Quarter Sessions to be held at a 'house of correction' as 'a foreigner' ... 'who is furiously mad'.[88]

When Thomas Mercer of Halstock, died in 1750, he was described as a physician in the burial register and a doctor in his will, and a detailed inventory was compiled and retained among his administration papers; his wife was named as Mary.[89] The document showed the assessment of his house and land which was valued at £35. Included in the inventory were: 'all his books and drugs £5', upwards of nine beds, seven dairy cows worth £25; a black gelding, hay racks and one stack of wheat. His given occupation and his stock of drugs reflected his primary occupation as a medical man, but he also maintained some agricultural interests, and the inventory reflects the Mercers' general prosperity. With a large number of beds in his household he may have cared for other residential patients besides Peter Bynen. An indication, perhaps, that the Mercer house in Halstock was operating as a private asylum under Thomas Mercer by the middle of the 18th century.

Thomas Mercer's first wife Mary had died in childbirth in 1732 and was buried on the same day their son Thomas was baptised. He married again, to another Mary, by 1735 and they had two sons, John and Justinian born in 1736 and 1739.[90] The three boys were 18, 14 and 11 years old when their father died in 1750, so it seems likely that only Thomas, the eldest, would have gained some medical experience or knowledge from their father. But, together with Mary, his widow, it is possible that the family continued to provide care for the insane within the parish. John's progress in the profession is not recorded. Justinian Mercer, the younger brother, was apprenticed for seven years to Oliver Hoskins, surgeon of Beaminster, in 1757 when he was 18 years old.[91] Apprenticeships usually began at around the age of 14, so the relatively late apprenticeship of Justinian may indicate that he had already gained some experience in the profession, perhaps alongside his mother and half-brother.[92]

In 1773 Justinian Mercer was described as an apothecary when he and Thomas Mercer, labourer, both of Halstock, pleaded guilty of an assault

88   DHC, Q/S/M/1/8.

89   WSHC, P5/1750/25.

90   DHC, PE-HAL/RE/1/1.

91   TNA, IR1/21, 1757.

92   For age of apprentices see for instance Levene, 'Parish apprenticeship', 915-41.

on Thomas Bartlett, gentleman and were fined 6*d.* at the Quarter Sessions.[93] However, it appears the fine was not paid and they were discharged. Justinian's training had led him to be described as an apothecary, a lower status than a surgeon, but still a trained medical man. The court case does not appear to have affected his future application to become proprietor of the asylum. The assault does not seem to be representative of the general character of the family who were most frequently recorded as pillars of the community. Generations of the Mercer family were active in the parish and evidently held in some regard by their peers. In 1744 and 1755 a John Mercer, victualler, appeared in the alehouse licence records.[94] Possibly the same John was acting as parish clerk, the earliest surviving churchwarden accounts record a salary payment of £1 for his 'clarkship' and for 'washing the surplice and cleaning the plate' he received 3*s.*; a position he continued for seven years (1759 -1766). Following his death in 1766 his son, Robert, continued the role which included 'bell ringing'.[95]

Other members of the family were resident in the same parish and the family was wholly integrated into the community. John Mercer and his wife Lydia were in business making articles of women's clothing, more particularly mantua gowns. John and Lydia, married 1743, were both recorded in apprenticeship registers as masters in the trade, first John in 1752[96] and later Lydia in 1777.[97] Ann Mercer, possibly their daughter-in-law, was master of the same trade to apprentices Edith Little in 1783,[98] and Mary Tarzawell in 1789.[99]

The brief glimpses of Thomas Mercer and his sons having trained as physicians and surgeons herald the beginning of the Halstock asylums and their long association with the Mercer family.

93 DHC, Q/S/M/2/9.
94 DHC, Q/D/L(V)/1/26 & 1/36.
95 DHC, PE-HAL/CW/1/1.
96 TNA, IR1/19, 1752.
97 TNA, IR1/29, 1777.
98 TNA, IR1/32, 1783.
99 TNA, IR1/65, 1789.

PRIVATE LICENCED ASYLUMS,
1774-1828

T HE ACT FOR Regulating Private Madhouses passed in 1774 required that all new and existing asylums should be licenced by the county Quarter Sessions. From this date some official records were maintained of all private houses that contained more than one inmate. In Dorset only the asylum at Halstock required a licence for an existing house, Stockland would apply for a licence for the first time in 1820.

The County Asylums Act of 1808, which enabled counties to establish public asylums, had little effect on the Dorset asylums as it did not trigger an immediate response within the county. So, there were no major changes to the management or oversight of Halstock or Stockland until the County Asylums Act of 1828 granted greater powers to visiting inspectors who also acquired to ability to close asylums in extreme circumstances.

Fees in respect of private patients were variable, relating to levels of care and accommodation available or required at the time. Another factor for those relying on family money was, no doubt, the ability or willingness to pay which for many was for an undefined number of years. No records survive showing the pauper or private fees charged at Halstock or Stockland. In 1816 the Puddletown overseers were paying 12s. a week for basic board for pauper patients, it is likely that private patient fees were substantially higher. Fees charged across some of the better known private houses over the same period varied between one to four guineas a week.[100] Exclusive asylums such as Ticehurst in Surrey, 'for the wealthier classes', commanded fees which largely depended on the individual's needs, wishes and depth of pocket.[101]

Pauper patient fees were generally fixed so contracts could be made with their home parish officials and were usually exclusive of clothing and medicines though this could also vary. As an example Laverstock House, a

100   Parry-Jones, *The Trade in Lunacy*, p.125.
101   Ibid., p.119.

private asylum in Fisherton Anger, Wiltshire, charged between 12s. and 14s. per week in 1815, without medicines.[102]

HALSTOCK

H ALSTOCK WAS HOME to the only Dorset asylum established before 1774. It was a small parish with a population of 397 in 1801 situated in the northwest of the county close to the Somerset border. Near neighbours were the villages of East Chelborough, Corscombe and Evershot and close towns were Sherborne and Yeovil. In 1836 it became part of the Beaminster Poor Law Union. In 1873 it was said to have been a healthy and thriving parish with 'no epidemic sickness having prevailed for upwards of forty years'.[103] It benefitted from the 'purest spring water' and the soil was noted to have been 'particularly favourable to the growth of oak'. It was a farming community with all the expected trades associated with a Dorset village in the early 19th century.

Under the Act for Regulating Private Madhouses two local Justices of the Peace, a physician and a Clerk of the Peace inspected Halstock asylum quite consistently and over long periods of time. The first Justice of the Peace was John Vincent who served for eight years until 1783 alongside Cuthbert Johnson, the physician and John Wallis, clerk, both of whom attended the asylum for 15 years. Overlapping these early years was Thomas Fox, rector of Wootton Glanville and Henry Sherive, Doctor of Law; they both visited for around 14 years. Perhaps the constancy of the Visitors provided a relatively helpful approach of long term oversight; it also provided a regular income for all concerned.

During the period 1774 to 1800 the visits occurred annually, except for 1783 when an additional inspection was made.[104] These visits were very likely unannounced and irregular. No reports appear in the Quarter Session records for 1776, 1777 and 1778 though there was an account record for 1776 where an inspection was apparently made by John Vincent, Justice of the Peace, who was paid £2 2s. 0d. and Cuthbert Johnson, the physician, whose remuneration was not recorded. From 1791 the Justices of the Peace each received £2 2s. 3d. for their trouble and the higher rate of £3 3s. 3d. was paid equally to the physician and clerk. The accounts also show two further

102   Ibid., p.126.
103   Hutchins, *History of Dorset,* III, p.465.
104   Q/A/L/Private/1.

payments made to the Secretary of the Quarter Sessions; one payment of
13s. 4d. for sending the details to the College of Physicians and a second
payment for their bill of expenses, £3 0s. 5d., for 'ordinaries & extraordinaries
for the days attendance (servants included).

Visitors received reimbursement for various expenses and the first of
these was recorded for 1779 'gave the servants of the said Messrs Mercers
agreeable to the directions of the said Mr Vincent and Fox, 8 shillings'. In
September 1782 a bill of expenses was paid by the court for 'the Silent Woman
for ordinarys and extraordinarys, servants included, as by bill of particulars' £1
13s. 2d.[105] The annual payments continued for such costs as in 1824, to William
Oglander, Justice of the Peace for 'car hire expenses at the inn, servants, etc.,
£1 2s. 6d.' and the same the following year to the Clerk. By 1827 expenses
had increased slightly to £1 5s. 0d. for 'car hire and expenses at the inn for Dr
Cooper and Mr Colson and self and also for the servants, horses, etc.'

The fee of 13s. 4d. was clearly paid even when a visit was not fulfilled
as can be seen from the account entry for the 19 May 1783

> my journey and horse hire to Maiden Newton on my way to Halstock
> agreeable to Mr Vincent's letter of the 4th instant to have met the Justices,
> but the weather proving very wet, and from the uncertainty of meeting
> gentlemen there, I waited the event of the weather and returned home.

He also submitted expenses for dinner of 4s. 4d. It appeared that the visit
took place instead the following day with the usual Visitors and included
expenses of £2.19s. 6d. at the Silent Woman. The secretary, John Wallis
recorded his fee of £3 3s. 0d. with details of his journey being '18 miles and
upwards' from Dorchester. A second visit was recorded in September 1783;
the first time this had occurred during this period. Perhaps this was due to
the merger of the two asylums newly under the care of Justinian Mercer. The
account continued with details of payments made to the four Visitors who
attended the asylum, and fees paid for sending a copy of the register minutes
of the proceedings and the usual expenses at the inn. The following year,
1784, reverted to just one inspection.

Visits to the asylum were often affected by adverse travelling
conditions, especially during the winter months; in the years 1775-1827
only around 10 visits took place across October, November December. Most
visits took place during more agreeable weather in springtime mostly from
May through the summer until September. Whilst good for the Visitors the

---

105   The Silent Woman was an inn in Halstock later known as The Quiet Woman.

Quarter Session account record showing payments made to John Vincent, the Visiting Justice; Dr Cooper, surgeon; Thomas Fox, clerk and John Wallis, their secretary, relating to their attendance to both asylum houses in Halstock, 1780 and 1781. Expenses are also shown for hospitality at the New Inn. DHC, Q/A/L.

situation relating to the patients during the colder months would have been largely unseen.

There were no annual visits recorded for 1792, 1793, 1803, 1807 and 1808 neither were entries made in the accounts. After 1810 only one Justice of the Peace carried out the annual inspection together with the usual physician and clerk. By 1827 Dr Cooper's fee had risen to £5 5s. 0d., the fee of the secretary Mr Fox remained at £3 3s. 0d. and the cost of transmitting the copy of the report was recorded at £1 1s. 0d. Further costs of £1 5s. 0d. were paid for the usual expenses. The Mercer family paid an annual fee of £10 and £15 to the court according to the number of patients expected to be confined for the coming year. This fee was payable regardless of the actual patient numbers. It seems unlikely that this fee alone completely covered the costs of the inspections, any overspend was probably subsidised by the court.

In their capacity as Justices of the Peace clergymen featured heavily in the visiting of the asylum across the next 50 or so years to 1828. The clergy Justices were Nathaniel Bristed, Morgan Jones, John Munden, Houlton Hartwell, John Morton Colson, John Vincent, esq. Members of the gentry were also appointed by the court as Justices of the Peace, two of which were Sir John Wyldbore Smith, baronet and Sir William Oglander, baronet. There were also members of parliament, including Francis John Browne of Frampton; he was known to have been an active and useful magistrate in Dorset.[106] Browne, who had no children, eventually gave his manor house at Forston to the county in order to establish a public asylum.

Under the provisions of the Act for Regulating Private Madhouses and, following applications made to the court, the brothers John and Justinian Mercer were each awarded a licence at a cost of £10 for the 'Reception of ten lunatics for the space of one year' in 1774. It was noted that they had for 'many years past kept a house for the reception of lunatics' within the parish. They now applied for two separate licences, for two distinct premises, although the licences did not state where the facilities managed by each brother were located.

Although the location of the two Madhouses was not recorded in the licences one was thought to be in an area known as Portland to the east of the village. The other may have been at Church House or possibly at a property facing the village green which, in later churchwarden accounts, can be identified as owned over the years by several members of the Mercer family.[107]

106 Thorne, 'Francis John Browne'.

107 DHC, PE-HAL/CW/1/1.

The Account of John Wallis of Dorchester in the
all Moneys by him received from Time to Time and of all
of an Act of Parliament made and passed in the Fourteenth
an Act for Regulating Madhouses Viz.

Accountant Dr.

1774 Nov. 19th	Receed of Mr. John Mercer of Halstock Surgeon for his Lycense granted him Bridport Sessions held the 4 Day of October 1774 pursuant to the above Statute as by my Receipt given him — — — — — —	£	10	0	0
	Ditto of Mr. Justinian Mercer of the same Place Surgeon as by my Receipt given him — — — —		10	0	0
1775 October 4	Ditto of Mr. John Mercer for his Lycense granted him Bridport Sessions held the 3 October 1775 for the Ensuing Year pursuant to the above Statute as by my Receipt given him — — — — —		10	0	0
	Ditto of Mr. Justinian Mercer for the like as by my Receipt given him — — — —		10	0	0
1776 October 9th	Ditto of Mr. John Mercer for his Lycense granted him Bridport Sessions held the 8th October 1776 for the Ensuing Year pursuant to the above Statute as by my Receipt given him — —		10	0	0
	Ditto of Mr. Justinian Mercer for the like as by my Receipt given him —		10	0	0
1777 October 7th	Ditto of Mr. John Mercer for his Lycense granted him Bridport Sessions held 7th October 1777 for the Ensuing Year pursuant to the above Statute as by my Receipt given him —		10	0	0
	Ditto of Mr. Justinian Mercer for the like as by my Receipt given him — — —		10	0	0
		£	80	0	0

Quarter Session account created by John Wallis, clerk, recording annual licence payments received from John and Justinian Mercer, 1774 to 1777. DHC, Q/A/L.

Halstock licence application 1774. DHC, Q/A/L.

Portland House was owned by John Pretor Pinney of Somerton Erle, who also owned considerable estates in the West Indies. The asylum and associated property which he leased to the Mercer family also provided accommodation for one of his sons and one of his employees. His son Pretor Pinney, born in Nevis in the West Indies, was buried at Halstock, aged 47, in May 1829. He had been a patient at the asylum for 20 years and at the time of his death the extensive family lands in Halstock had passed to his older brother John F. Pinney. The second patient at Halstock with links to John Pretor Pinney was Joseph Gill, a one time sugar plantation manager on Nevis. He was listed in the asylum register once in 1787, aged 35, but later discharged at an unknown date. He returned to Halstock in

1797 to board with Christopher Guppy, the tenant of the agricultural lands at Portland Farm.[108]

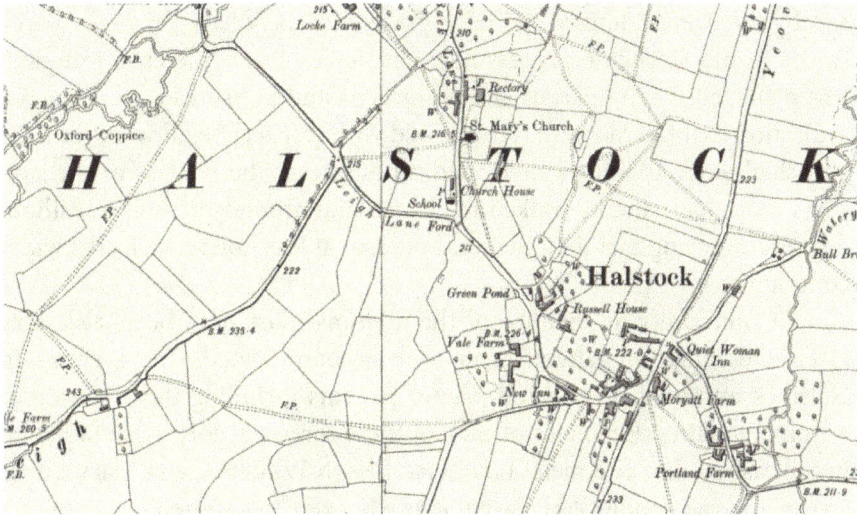

Ordnance Survey map of Halstock, 1903.

Joseph Gill appears to have been highly regarded by John Pretor Pinney who remembered him in his will where he was described as 'Joseph Gill living at Portland Farm, Halstock'. In the bequest he was to be furnished with a complete set of mourning clothes and John F. Pinney erected a memorial to him in the parish church, in contrast to his brother whose grave at the church is unmarked.[109] Although no leases have been located, it is possible that the Mercer family's long tenancy of Portland Farm was linked to their relationship with the Pinney family.

The limits on the number of patients allowed was a key provision of the Act for Regulating Private Madhouses, 1774; the fee was set at £10 for any number not exceeding ten patients. Asylums housing in excess of ten patients were to incur a charge of £15, with no apparent upper limit to the number they could accommodate. From 1801 the court record relating to Justinian Mercer's asylum ceased to specify the number of lunatics within his application and more than ten were regularly present. The need for places was high; 23 patients were in residence in 1812, and of these eight were occupied by paupers.

108   C. Eikelmann, *The Mountravers Plantation Community*, part 2, chapter 4, p.420. (website accessed 26 August 2025).

109   TNA, PROB 11/1605/155.

How the presence of the two newly licenced asylums was received by the community is unknown. They were not mentioned in contemporary church records and the court documents do not offer any insight. An asylum run by the Mercer family had been present in the village for many years, so the formal licencing process may have made little difference to how it was managed. Their roles as churchwardens and parish clerks provide an indication that the Mercer's were viewed with respect, well known for their parochial work as well as their medical business. The records in the later years note that patients walked to church and around the village without incident; showing that they were accepted, or at least tolerated, by the wider community.

Community acceptance of the asylums must have been necessary given the range of patients who were accommodated. The asylums in Halstock admitted private and pauper patients including those classed as criminal lunatics. Examples of each of these three categories can be found in the case studies of Amelia Lindquist, Joseph Whiterow and Mary Curtis (see below, case studies). Those patients who were transferred to an asylum, rather than being maintained in cheaper locations such as parish lodgings, the family home or the workhouse were generally those who might be more disruptive.

John and Justinian continued to run their respective asylums until 1781 when John Mercer died aged 45. His mother, now remarried and known as Mary Esgar, obtained a licence to continue managing John's asylum until her death two years later.[110] Her willingness to take on the business suggests that she had also been partly responsible for its survival (prior to licencing in 1774) when her children were both minors. The Quarter Sessions certainly took the view that she was a suitable person to take on the licence. Following Mary's death in both asylums were joined together under the proprietorship of her surviving son, Justinian.

A period of relative stability followed until Justinian Mercer's death in 1810, at the age of 72.[111] The asylum was then taken on by his son-in-law John Mercer, married to Justinian's daughter Alice. John, born in 1783 to Thomas and Ann Mercer, had gained his surgeon status through his apprenticeship to his grand-father Justinian which commenced in 1805.[112] John was just 22 years old when he took over the asylum. A Thomas Mercer, probably his father, was noted in the Quarter Session Order books as a guarantor in

110   DHC, Q/S/M/1/10, f. 418.

111   DHC, PE-HAL/RE/1/2.

112   TNA, R1/40.

Register of patients under the care of Justinian Mercer at Halstock asylum, August 1800. Details of age, occupation and place of abode is shown for almost all those listed with three people identified as paupers. DHC, Q/A/L.

the form of a 'Recognizance' for £100 which related to the asylum licence application together with John Mercer in 1813.[113]

During the later 18th and early 19th centuries the Mercer family maintained their position as stalwart members of Halstock society. Between 1778 and 1781 Justinian Mercer, apothecary, was a signatory to the minutes of the vestry meetings. In 1815 another Justinian Mercer, likely to be the son of Thomas and Ann, of was listed as a 'proprietor and occupier' in a church rate made for the repair and support of the parish church of Halstock. His assessment was low on the list at 2d.[114] There was some overlap between the family's parish duties and their medical business. In March 1815 Thomas Mercer was signatory to the minutes of the vestry meeting and in the same year the overseers' account noted that Dr John Mercer agreed to 'take the medical care of the poor for the year' for a payment of

113   DHC, Q/S/M/1/14, f.61.

114   DHC, PE-HAL/CW/1/1.

£10 which was repeated in April 1816. Dr Mercer would be responsible for general medical matters, except for resetting compound fractures and administering vaccinations. He attended a patient the following year for which he received £2 for services. In 1818 his medical care continued, the vestry was again in agreement that he was paid £10 a year. This contract included responsibilities for parishioners taken ill elsewhere and he was to receive addition compensation for attending to them.

In 1818 John Mercer died aged 34. His widow Alice and her sister Betsy Mercer, the daughters of Justinian and Grace Mercer, continued the business and made known their intention to carry on 'their long established Lunatic Asylum at Halstock' in the usual way through an advertisement in the local newspaper.[115] They were keen to reassure people that a surgeon of 'considerable experience and who is Member of the College of Surgeons in London attends the house almost daily'. This surgeon may have been Dr Thomas Shorland who took over John Mercer's contract with the parish to attend to the poor with general medical care.[116] The sisters requested that anyone with claims on his estate should advise Mrs Mercer so they may be discharged. Similarly, those indebted to the late John Mercer were requested to settle.

Little is known about the two Mercer sisters and what drove them to continue managing the asylum through the decades. No family or business correspondence remains. Certainly, following the death of John Mercer in 1818 his widow, Alice, could have chosen a different path or supervised a much smaller property. The overseer accounts show that the poor relief, that had previously been paid by John Mercer, was now paid, in 1819, by Alice Mercer who was described as the proprietor and occupier of the family's unnamed property in the parish.[117] This may have been the property the family kept as their own, independent of the asylum; perhaps where they lived and on occasion cared for people such as Mrs Berkely, a patient, who was moved to live under the care of John Justinian Mercer's Aunt (Betsy) in 1839.

Conditions within the asylum at Halstock were rarely mentioned in the reports, but overcrowding was an issue that concerned the Visitors. To complicate this process there was also a concern regarding the mixing up of patients who are 'outrageous' with those who were considered to be

115   *Salisbury and Winchester Journal* (31 August 1818)
116   DHC, PE-HAL/OV/1.
117   Ibid.

'quiet and inoffensive', and a national concern to separate the sexes.[118] These concerns can be demonstrated at Halstock in the case of Amelia Lindquist who was removed because she proved to be too difficult to manage and was also found to be pregnant while in the asylum.[119] Yet, given the number of years the asylum was in business it is remarkable that this appears to be an isolated incident and any potential problems that might be caused by the mixing of patients with different requirements were probably resolved by other means.

Information collected about the patients and recorded in the Quarter Sessions varied year to year. During the first 25 years, 1775-1802, the court recorded patients' ages and occupations and drew a distinction between private patients and paupers (see Appendix 1). Given Halstock's proximity to its neighbouring county it is unsurprising that of the ten people listed in 1775 at John Mercer's asylum the majority were from Somerset, six in all. Another three were from Devon and only one from Dorset; two of the ten were paupers. Two were women and four men, the average age was 37; the eldest at 70 was Cain Andrews and the youngest George Hunt from Horsington, just 15 years old. Four years later he was still confined and after this time he disappears from the records.

The asylum belonging to the younger brother Justinian Mercer housed four people, two male and two female, three from Somerset and one from Dorset in 1775, their average age was 43. Two were paupers, Mrs Elizabeth Brown and Martin Pottle. Only basic information was recorded at this time: their name, place of abode, status or occupation and age, women were defined by their marital status.

From the outset two paupers were listed in Justinian Mercer's asylum. As the years progressed the Quarter Session register noted an increase of pauper patients. Asylums were not required to maintain an admission and discharge register, but patients were named in the report made at the time Visitor's inspection. Further records of patients no longer confined through either death or discharge was not a requirement of the Act in 1774. Consequently, patients disappeared from the asylum's records with no explanation. At Halstock a Mrs Margaret Drake was entered in the parish burial register in 1779 with the note that she was 'a patient at Justinian Mercer's'.[120] Neither she or another patient, George Tozer, buried in 1799, had been recorded in the records submitted to the Quarter Sessions. No

118   *First Report from the Committee on the State of Asylums* (1815).

119   see Case Studies, below.

120   DHC, PE-HAL/RE/1/2.

Halstock asylum's first register of 1775 recorded for the Quarter Session court lists the patients in the respective houses of John and Justinian Mercer. Collectively two of the ten patients are identified as paupers and one, George Hunt, is the youngest at 15 years of age. The report was made by the Visiting Justice, John Vincent, the surgeon, Cuthbert Johnson and their Secretary John Wallis. DHC, Q/A/L.

doubt there would have been others. These omissions could simply be the result of inadequate record keeping, but more likely to have been due to patients staying for short periods of time between official visits.

The Quarter Session reports in the early years reflected a decline in the numbers of patients from 14 in 1775 to just six in 1781 across both houses managed by John and Justinian Mercer. Clearly both were falling short of the ten people allowed in the terms of their individual licences. The numbers changed little as the years progressed, increasing to just nine patients by the end of the century. The asylum houses had been joined as one in 1783 and from 1797 the licence covered 15 patients.

In August 1800 the register recorded eleven patients: seven men and four women. Three were identified as paupers, the others comprised a wife, a gentleman, a Navy Lieutenant, a single woman, a currier and a widow. There were two from Somerset, four Devon and five Dorset. Some private patients came to Halstock from further afield. In 1809 a Miss Oakes from London was present in the asylum. There is no further information about her in the Quarter Sessions records or the parish registers, although there is a headstone for a Betsy Oakes in the Halstock churchyard dated 1810.[121] No official body required that deaths at the asylum should be reported at this time.

In the first decade of the 19th century recording of personal information was even more sporadic than in the previous century. Occupations and ages were largely overlooked with the occasional exception. Ages were again recorded from 1815 to 1819 but ceased to be noted in 1820. The usual places or residence of patients were only noted between 1820 and 1828.

From their earliest inspections the regular phrase used by the Visitors to describe what they regarded as satisfactory conditions was: 'all found to be in clean and decent apparel and well accommodated with all the necessaries of life'. The demeanour of the patients was regularly noted to be 'all tranquil and comfortable'. These stock phrases, contained in brief reports, provide no information about the conditions of individual patients.

The first recorded observation made regarding the health and state of a patient related to Sarah Noake. The Visitors in August 1802 noted in the margin of the register that they 'deem her only afflicted with a Mania Hysterica'. She does not appear in the register again and this was an isolated report with no observations relating to other patients. Although paupers were not always identified they could occasionally be distinguished from private patients who were often afforded titles, such as Mr or Mrs. Those cured or those no longer confined for other reasons remained unrecorded.

Prior to the Madhouse Act 1828, across a time span of 53 years, little appears to have changed in the management and treatment of the patients at Halstock asylum. The Visitors continued to make their inspections and to document all that was required of them. If the Justices of the Peace, clerks and physicians had knowledge about treatment and care this was not shared with the court, there was no legal need. In the final report of March 1828, before the new legislation, virtually the same observation was being relayed as it had since the earliest assessment:

121   DHC, *Parish transcript* (No.51).

'... and of the patients therein confined we have found them all lunatics and is as clean a situation as their cases will admit and that the house is in all respects proper and fit for such reception and purpose being situate in an exceeding healthy country and without any cause of complaint'. Colson and Cooper MD.

Like treatment, cure and the nature of illness and death, other aspects of daily life and activities were scarcely mentioned. There was some kitchen work, reading and needlework, occasional engagement with music, but still with little or no reported opportunity for meaningful employment. On a rare occasion in 1822, the Visitors found Robert Gould, a private patient, to be absent from the asylum having 'gone on a visit to Evershott'. He was later seen at the inn by Dr Cooper. In contrast, discussion around activities for pauper patients, or anyone thought 'difficult', was not reported; it is likely that their activity was restricted to a short spell outside in the designated walled areas.

Halstock asylum ran continuously for 84 years in which time there were relatively few serious incidents which were made known to the visiting magistrates. The story of Amelia Lindquist is discussed in the cases studies (see below). Another serious incident was a dual escape made through the roof of the asylum by Thomas Barrett, a blacksmith from Frampton and Samuel Hopkins of Milton Abbas which was reported in May 1821 when they had not yet been been found. A year later Thomas Barrett had returned and appeared in the asylum register but Samuel Hopkins remained at large it seems as he was not spoken of again. Barrett, originally confined in 1815, was 'very desirous of his liberty'. The Visitors recommended that he should be allowed to go to church and suggested that the visiting surgeon needed to pay attention to the state of his mind. In 1832 he was admitted to Forston asylum aged 74. His order paper described him as married with eight children, that he could be violent at times and was fond of drinking; his cause of insanity was not known.[122] He was buried in his home parish of Frampton in 1841 aged 82.[123]

The only suicide at Halstock was reported occurred in May 1829. Joseph Foss, a fisherman from Chideock, had been in the asylum for just over a month when he made his escape. A search was made within ten minutes of his absence being noticed, but his body was not found until

122   DHC, NG-HH/CMR/4/32A/021.

123   DHC, PE-FRA/RE/4/1.

several days later. The Visitors, in November 1829, were critical of the proprietor of the asylum, Alice Mercer, for allowing him to have free use of his hands knowing that he was vulnerable to self harm.

The tragedy was recorded in the *Bath Chronicle and Weekly Gazetteer*, 11 June 1829:

A man named Joseph Foss, of Chideock, near Bridport, confined at Halstock Lunatic Asylum, Dorset, contrived to elude the vigilance of his keepers about a fortnight since, and, after an ineffectual search, was discovered accidentally by a shepherd boy, in a hedge, a few miles from Halstock, with a portion of rope round his neck, and another portion attached to a stump in the hedge. It appears that in his effort to destroy himself, the rope had broken but the pressure was such as to occasion death. He was in such a state when found, that it became difficult to remove his clothes, and he was interred with them on at Chideock.

Despite these occasional incidents, the overall the impression of the Halstock asylum in the period 1774-1828 is one of a relatively well managed institution which had managed to recover from the death of John Mercer in 1818 and was run by his widow to a standard accepted by the Visitors.

STOCKLAND

D ORSET'S SECOND PRIVATE asylum could be found in the small parish of Stockland which was chiefly a farming community in the east of the county. It was transferred from Dorset to Devon in 1844. John Hutchins in his *History of Dorset* described Stockland abounding with high hills and deep valleys, remarkably healthy and considered the situation to be 'romantic'. He noted that the soil 'is chiefly a stiff glutinous red clay, that bears good crops of wheat and oats, and is very fit for potter's ware and making brick', he also recognised its 'excellent springs'. The land was used mainly for dairy farming, arable, sheep pasture and for the growth of furze and peat for fuel.[124] Over half of the inhabitants were employed in agriculture.[125]

This open landscape of rolling hills and scattered dairy farms was considered by contemporaries to be an ideal location for an asylum. The *Sherborne Mercury* published the following in 1821:

124   Hutchins, *History of Dorset*, II, p.246.

125   Industry statistics, 1800-1831, www.visionofbritain.org.uk/ (website accessed 26 August 2025)

A serious gentleman lately made the following remarks on his Topographical Tour through the West of England, which, for their peculiar apposite description, just and appetible sensibility of expression, admirably calculated for the amelioration the most wretched of the Human Species, are deserving of publication: - Passing along the great spacious arrow-road on the summit of Stockland Hill, from the Devonshire Inn, to Seaton, he saw the direction Mr Spicer's Asylum at Boardhays, for Maniacs; and attracted by the expansive magnificent scenery of Land and Sea views, he exclaimed, in a kind of rapture, "What a choice spot for an Asylum of this sort. The best I have ever seen, simple and rural amusements, beautiful, humble, exhilarating, and sublime attractions, aided by salubrious Sea and Land breezes, all conspiring to awaken exquisite pleasure in the most pensive mind, and tending, as it were, by Panacea of Nature, to sooth the paroxysms of the most deranged faculties into complacency.[126]

The asylum was officially established and licenced by 1820 by William Clarke Spicer who remained the proprietor until its closure in 1841. A recognisance fee of £100 was noted for William Clarke Spicer, surgeon, and Thomas Dean, gentleman, of Chardstock £100. Two Justices of the Peace William Tucker, esq., and Francis Goforth, clerk, were appointed as future Visitors along with physician Dr Robertson of Honiton.[127]

Spicer was born in Chard in 1786, to parents William Clarke and Susannah, and baptised there, aged 8, together with his brother, Northcote, in 1794.[128] His father's occupation, as stated in his will, was surgeon and apprenticeship documents showed him as 'master' to apprentice Thomas Palmer in Chard,1794. Both William and Northcote followed their father in his profession and became surgeons. William, as the eldest son, received the bulk of his father's substantial estate which was to be bequeathed to his children after his death in 1820.[129]

William Clarke Spicer married Mary Broughton by licence in January 1811 in Wambrook about two miles from Chard, although his residence at the time was given as Membury in Devon.[130] An earlier record showed a marriage bond between William Clarke of Membury, yeoman and Mary of

126   *Sherborne Mercury,* 5 March 1821.
127   DHC, Q/S/M/1/15, f.42.
128   SHC, D/P/CHARD 2/1/2.
129   TNA, PROB/11/1630/11.
130   SHC, D/P/WAM/2/1/4.

Wambrook officiated by the Dean of Sarum in 1810.[131] The couple had nine children. Their father was described as a gentleman when first born son William Clarke Spicer was baptised in 1811. The children's father continued to be described as such until the baptisms of his two of sons in 1832, when the register recorded him as keeper of the asylum at Boardhays.[132]

Early documented reference to Spicer's involvement in the lunacy business remains elusive. The parish register described him as a keeper of the asylum in 1816 four years before he was granted a licence by the Quarter Sessions. It was not uncommon for surgeons to provide accommodation for one or two lunatics, so perhaps he did so within his home before he applied for official status as an asylum keeper in 1820. Land tax returns of 1827 and 1828 suggest that he was occupier of Bursehays owned by the Revd Thomas Putt.[133] Perhaps this was the family home as it appears to be a different site to Boardhay's and Ford where the asylum premises were licenced after 1828.

In the early years the asylum was known within the court records as Boardhay's or simply the 'asylum'. In October 1834 the Quarter Session

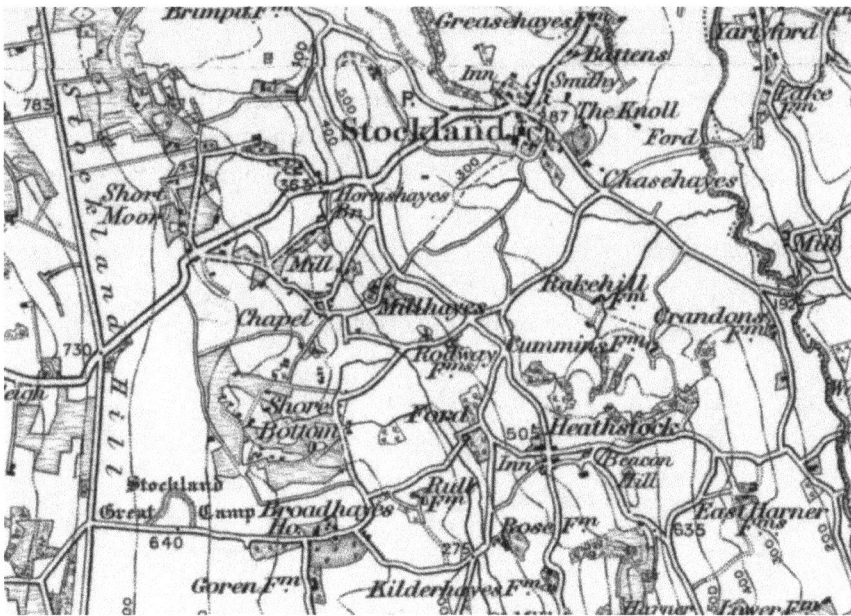

Ordnance Survey map of Stockland, 1898, showing Broadhayes (alias Boardhayes) and Ford to the south of the village.

131   WSHC, D1/62/4.
132   DvnHC,1215A/PR/1/3.
133   DHC, Q/D/E(L)/59/40-5.

Order book referred to the asylum as 'Ford' at the time of licence renewal.[134] No record was made of the asylum relocating to different premises which suggests that the change was made in name only. The property was situated within easy reach of the village, by lanes and footpaths and importantly, the church at only a mile or so distance.

Following its establishment in 1820 licences covering the asylum's first two years were granted for ten patients. The number was unspecified between 1822 and 1828 by which time it had been increased to 25.[135] Although Spicer was awarded his initial licence in 1820 there were no annual visits minuted in the court records until 1828. During these years licences were granted as the court accounts confirm payments made by Spicer from 1820 to 1823 at £10 and £15 for the years 1824 to 1827, indicating that the number of patients for which the asylum was licenced had been increased to 25 in 1824. No fees for the Visitors were entered into the accounts payable before 1828, so it seems likely that the asylum was not visited during its first eight years.

Patient records were not well kept at Stockland therefore the survival of information relating to patient numbers is limited to the years 1820, 1822-1823, 1830-1833 and 1836-1837 (see Appendix 1). It was a slow start, just two private patients were recorded from 1820 and the first two pauper patients arrived in 1822. Pauper patient numbers jumped substantially the following year with fifteen men and five women joining the two male and two female private patients. It appears that in 1823 Spicer chose to shift his professional interests from being a surgeon who maintained a small number of patients in his home to concentrating on managing the asylum as his main business with a primary focus of accommodating pauper patients.

---

134   DHC, Q/S/M/1/16.

135   DHC, Q/S/M/1/15 -1/16.

PRIVATE ASYLUMS AND THE NEW
COUNTY ASYLUM, 1828 -1842

THE COUNTY ASYLUMS Act, 1828 (known as the Madhouse Act)
strengthened the powers available to the Visitors. From 1828 to 1842
the Dorset Justices included one member of Parliament, Robert Gordon,
who was also a Metropolitan Commissioner. He later became one of
the unpaid Lunacy Commissioners and was known to have been one of
the most active honorary commissioners second only to the 7th Earl of
Shaftesbury. The clerical Justices were John White, John Parsons and W.
J. Goodden. Other Justices appointed as Visitors included Henry Digby, a
senior Royal Navy officer who had inherited the Minterne Magna estate in
Dorset from his uncle Admiral Robert Digby, Samuel Pretor, a banker and
tenant of the Digby's Sherborne House, and Samuel Cox, Justice of the
Peace, Deputy Lieutenant and chair of Beaminster Board of Guardians.

Robert Gordon was probably the most knowledgeable and qualified
in respect of the lunacy 'business'. He had visited Halstock twice in the
latter months of 1828. His Dorset property was Leweston House near
Sherborne; he was member of Parliament for Wareham, Cricklade and
New Windsor at various times from 1812 to 1841. Active on many issues,
he chaired select committee meetings in 1827 which he had brought
about following 'the dreadful state of misery' he had found in the keeping
of pauper patients in Middlesex. It was at his instigation that the 1828
Private Asylums Bill was introduced to Parliament for establishing public
asylums in the counties. He worked closely with the Earl of Shaftesbury
and their efforts to reform the care of lunatics placed Dorset at the centre
of these changes. He was a Commissioner in Lunacy until his death in
1864.[136]

The Madhouse Act 1828 called for the Visitor's to be vigilant of any
improper confinement of a patient. The issue of improper confinement
seems to have been a foremost priority for the Dorset Visiting Justices and

136 Thorne, 'Robert Gordon', *History of Parliament.*

was in marked contrast to the lack of attention paid to improving the lives of those incarcerated.[137]

HALSTOCK

THE 1828 ACT had an immediate effect within Dorset and in the second half of this noteworthy year Halstock was visited by three Justices of the Peace, a physician and a clerk on three occasions, having previously been visited once per year. This increased number of visits continued, averaging four times a year, until 1842. Usually, two or more Justices of the Peace visited the asylum, but on a handful of occasions inspections were made by just one Justice of the Peace along with the physician and clerk. It was a huge change to the annual assessment of the previous decades and had a considerable impact. Samuel Cox consistently visited the asylum at Halstock three to four times a year, almost without a break, for around 18 years.[138] The physician Samuel Bradley was also a constant presence, his attendance continued from 1828 to 1842.

The Act had also made provision for visits by friends of the lunatics every six months. the term was used to describe those who had been responsible for the patient's confinement and might include family, friends, overseers or clergymen. In December 1828 there had been three certificates of visits from friends issued at Halstock since last meeting which the legislation directed should be kept with the register.

An asylum the size of Halstock was required at this time to receive a visit from a medical man once or twice a week and keep a record of patient care. This Medical Journal was to include male and female numbers, those thought to be curable or otherwise and those under restraint. During previous years 1819 to 1828, under Alice Mercer, medical treatment had not been recorded. Now, as a result of the Act, the Visitors noted in December 1828 that 'the Weekly Register for the observations of the Medical attendant has been provided and appears to be correctly kept'.

The identity of the Medical Attendant was not usually stated though in 1828 the Visitors noted in reference to the care of Mrs Davis: 'Mr Shorland to attend to the bodily health of this lady'. The Shorland's were a family of eminent surgeons working in and around Yeovil. Thomas Shorland set up practice in the town with his son William in 1830 and both had a

---

137   Brown, *History of Dorset Hospitals*, p.161.
138   Hutchins, *History of Dorset*, v.4, p.169.

connection with the asylum working as doctors attending to the patients. In 1842 William was to become one of the court's appointed Visitors to the asylum.

In 1828 the asylum premises can be identified as a collection of buildings later known as Portland-on the eastern edge of Halstock village. They were owned by John F. Pinney and occupied by Alice Mercer until 1838 and then by her son, John Justinian Mercer, until his death in 1848.[139]

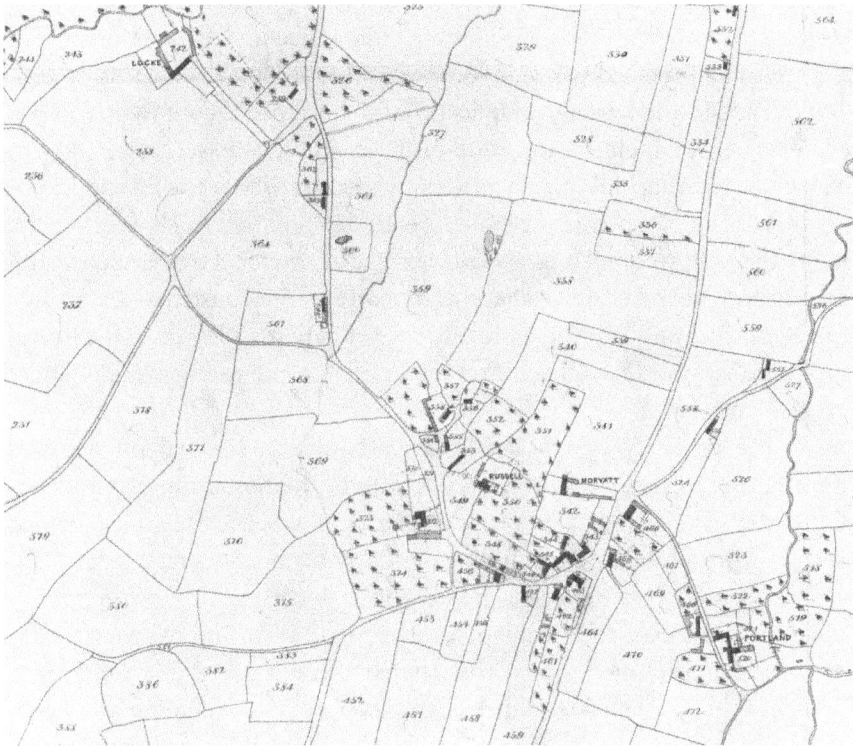

Section of the Halstock tithe map with accompanying apportionment created in 1845. The accompanying apportionment lists land and property connected to John Justinian Mercer including the asylum (number 520, marked 'Portland'). He owned the property numbered 344 in the centre of the village, a house with offices, garden and orchard in heart of village. This was probably where Robert Meredith lived in 1845 and where asylum moved to in 1849. Agricultural fields numbered 334, 464 and 483 were also owned and occupied by John Justinian. DHC, T/HAL.

The Tithe map of 1845 shows the position of the asylum and other Mercer properties. The asylum occupied an acre at Portland where the property was described in the tithe apportionment as *'house, offices &*

139   DHC, PE-HAL/CW/1/1

garden' rather than being identified as an 'asylum'. Although he leased Portland House, John Justinian Mercer owned a property in the centre of the village, a house, offices, garden and orchard of 0.5 acre which was leased to Revd Robert Meredith, pasture land of over 1.5 acres, running south of the village and two small pieces of agricultural land called 'Bit' pasture and Lyde Marsh meadow.

Under the terms of the 1828 Act asylum keepers were obliged to submit plans of their premises to the Quarter Sessions for approval by the committee of Visitors. Two letters from Alice and Betsy Mercer were addressed to Thomas Fooks, clerk of the peace for Dorset, dated April 1829. One relates to their licence application for no more than 25 patients and expressed their intention to reside in the house. It was accompanied by a plan of the existing building dated 1828. The second letter was an application for an Auxiliary House for six patients with the intention to 'superintend the same' and was accompanied by another plan. It appears that if the existing house and planned additional accommodation were constructed as shown, and both were fully occupied, the number of patients allowed in the licence applications would have been exceeded unless some rooms were intended for residential staff.

The property called 'Portland Cottage' was situated on a corner showing the main road from Yeovil to Sherborne bordering on two sides; another 'border' shows the Portland river from whence the area is named. The drawing presents the buildings and layout of the surrounding land including animal sheds, a brewhouse and stable. A section of the ground is defined for 'men; and 'women', an exercise area for the pauper inmates. Areas of land adjacent and across the road are marked as belonging to Colonel Pinney. The plan includes extensive grounds including a 'pleasure garden', 'lawn' and two 'kitchen gardens' which, if drawn with patient outdoor activity in mind, shows some knowledge and forward thinking on the part of the Mercer sisters.

The ground floor plan is detailed with a kitchen, pantry, beer cellar and a room set aside for a surgery. Two rooms are prescribed for the use of the 'Gentleman', a parlour and sitting room with a 'family sitting room' which presumably was for the use of the 'Ladies' and, perhaps, the Mercer family. One door lead outside to the 'Pleasure' garden and another to an area marked as 'Lawn'. The laundry and scullery areas were accessed separately from a small court.

The plan clearly shows the division of accommodation between the private and pauper patients. There were two rooms reserved for the 'women'

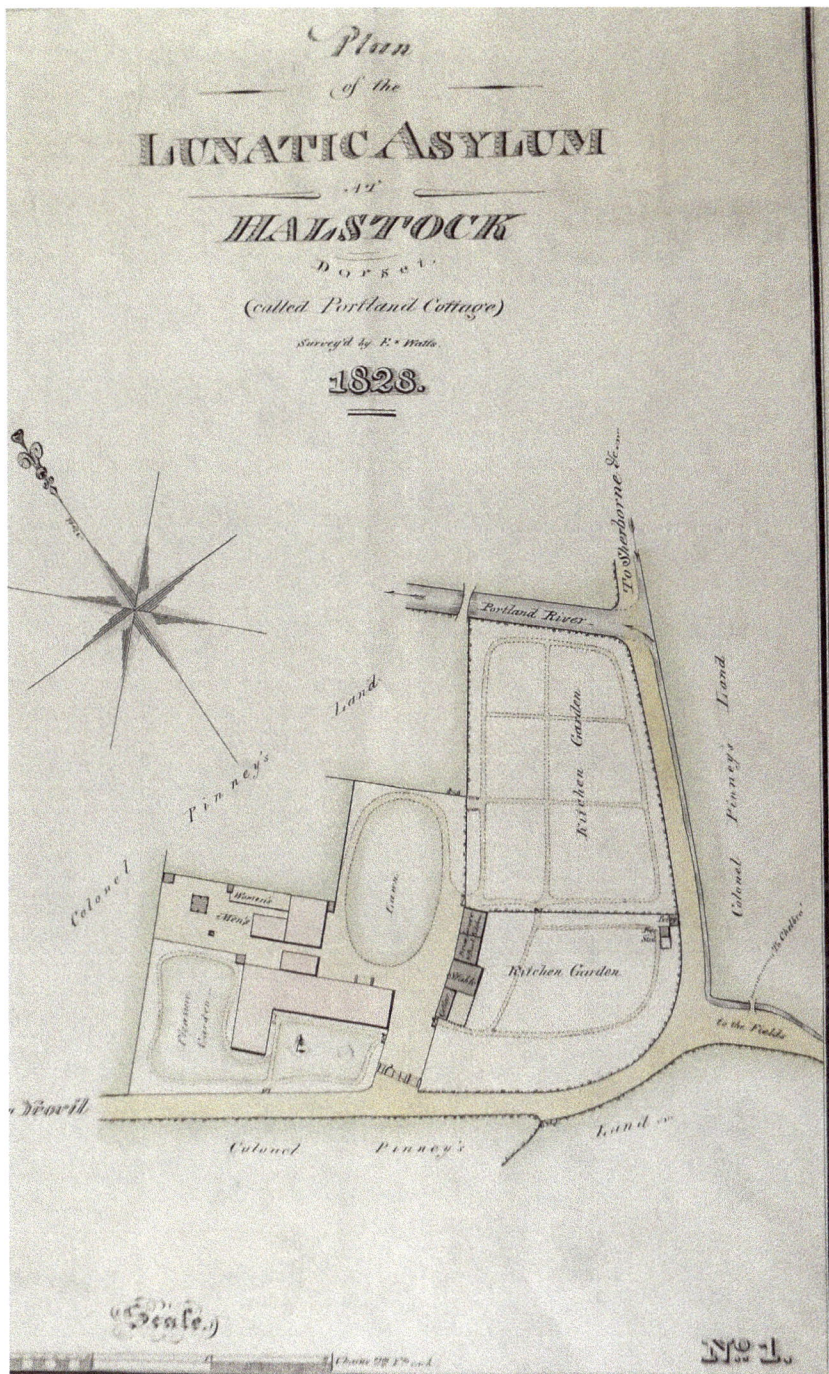

Halstock asylum, identified as Portland Cottage, bird's eye plan produced to accompany licence application, plan no.1. 1828. DHC, Q/A/L.

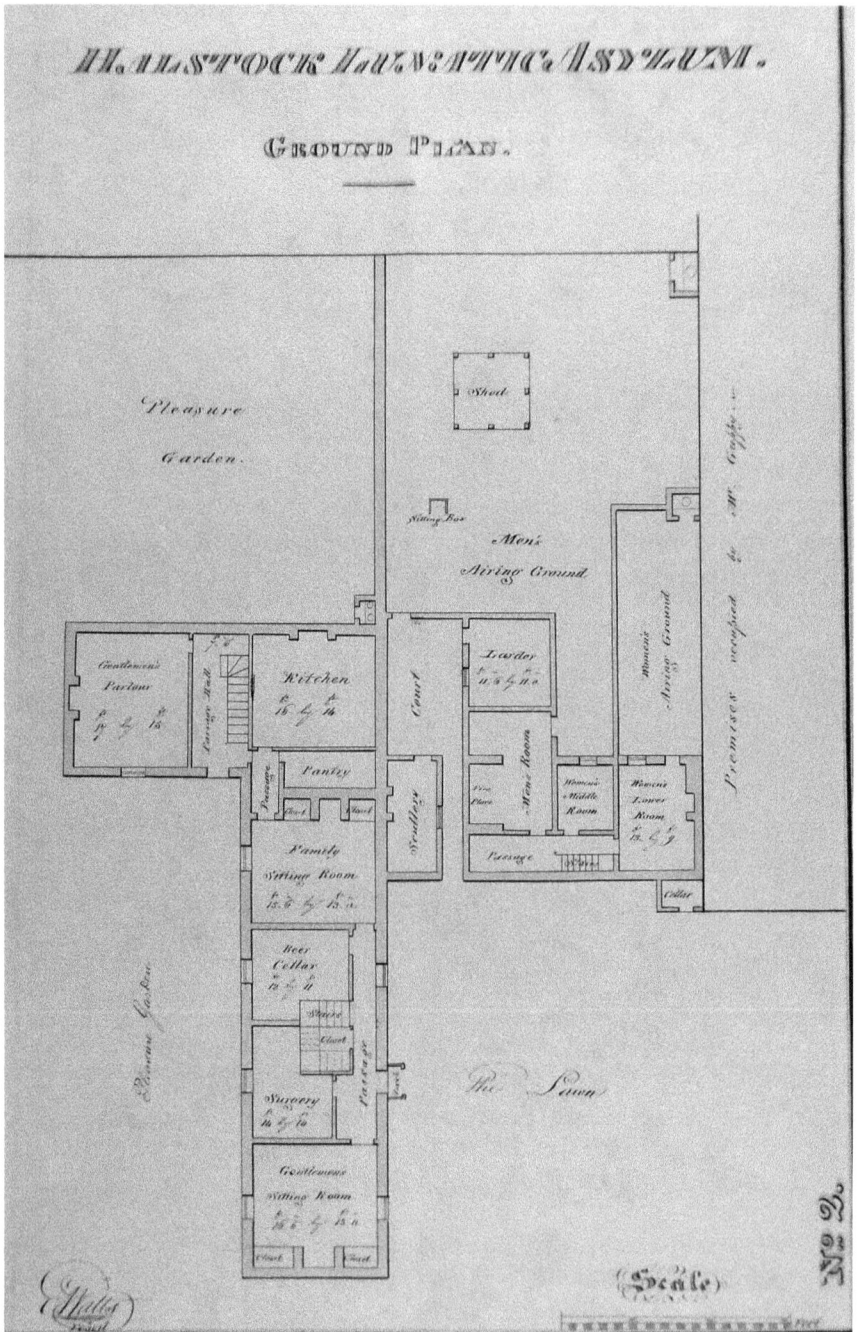

Halstock, ground floor plan, plan no. 2. 1828. DHC, Q/A/L.

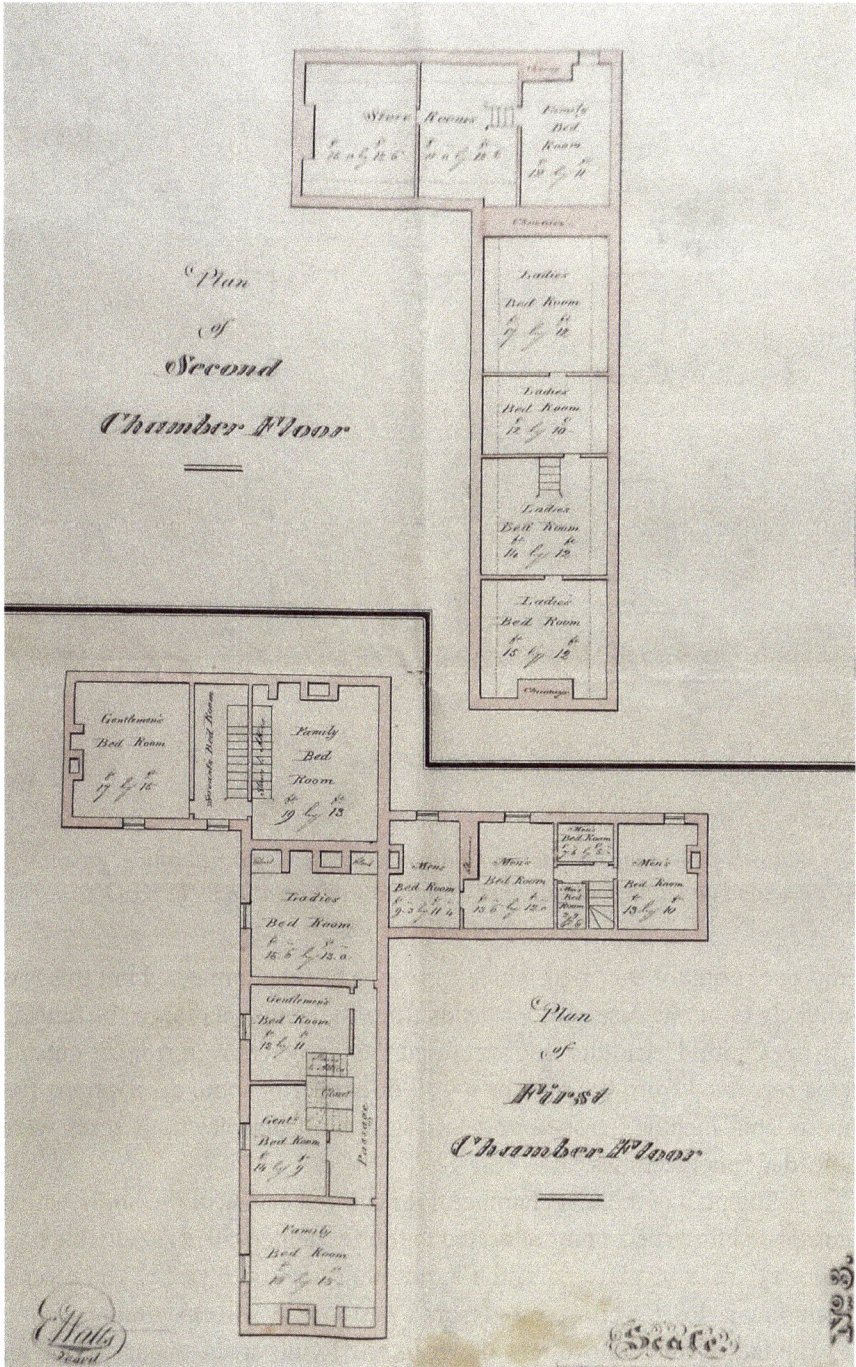

Halstock, 1st and second floors, plan no.3. 1828. DHC, Q/A/L

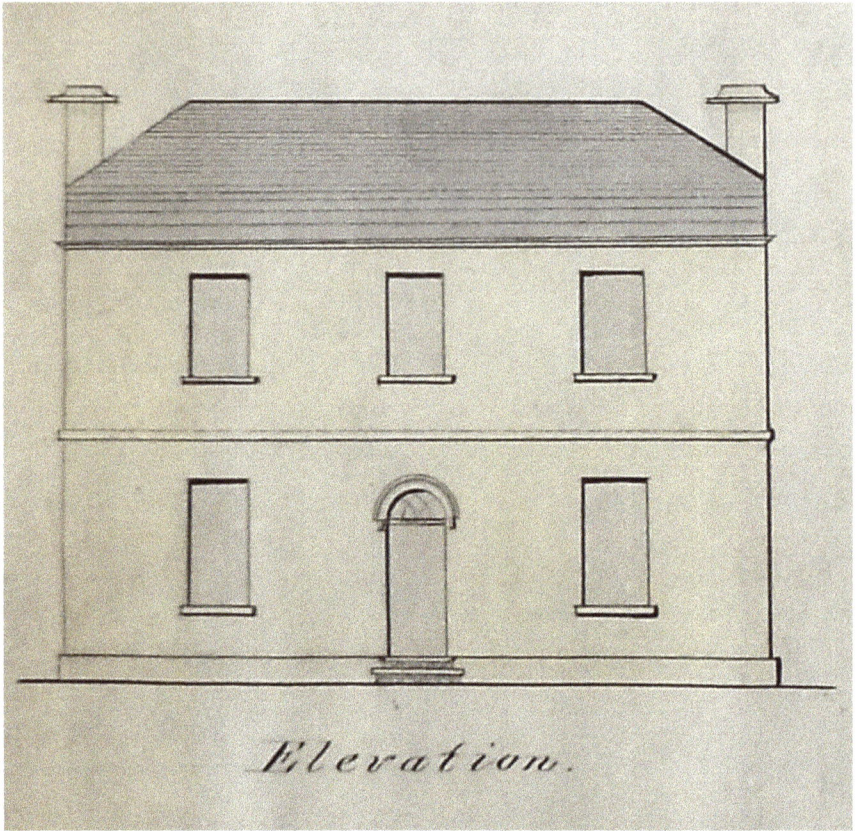

Halstock, plan of the intended auxiliary asylum showing the elevation, ground, second and attic floors together with the outside area, 1829. DHC, Q/A/L (continued next page).

and one room for the 'men' which appear to be interconnected but this was unlikely to be the case. A door; leads from the men's section to the outside 'Airing Ground'. Another door accessed the women's much smaller outside area separated from the men by a wall or barrier of some description. The men's area included a shed and 'sitting box'; it appears both sexes were afforded toilet facilities.

The plan of the first chamber floor showed a wing of the house which comprised three bedrooms allocated to the gentlemen, all of reasonable size: 16' x 13', 14' x 9', 12' x 11' and a ladies bedroom 15' 6" x 13'. The rooms, including a closet, were accessed from a passageway with a staircase leading to the ladies floor above and down to the living areas. Separated by an internal wall there were a further two bedrooms, one measuring 17' x 15' was assigned for a gentleman and across the landing a family bedroom 19' x

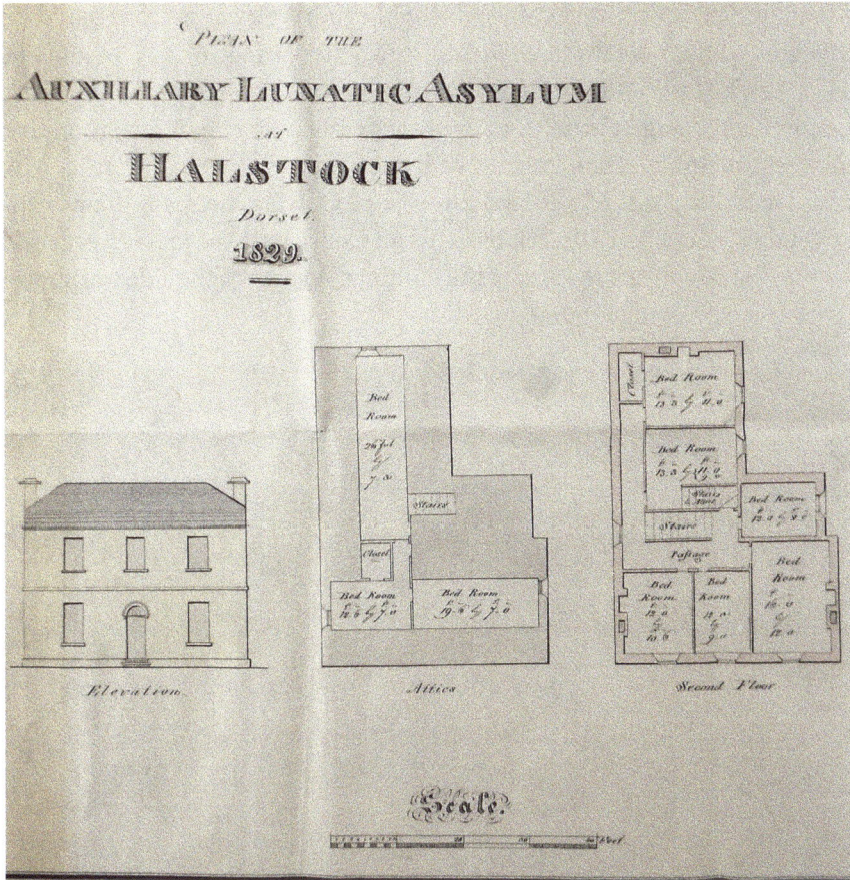

'PLAN OF THE
AUXILIARY LUNATIC ASYLUM
at
HALSTOCK
Dorset
1829

Elevation. Attica. Second Floor.

Scale.

13'. In between these two rooms there was a small servants' bedroom which included a staircase which led to the ground floor and ladies bedrooms above. On the same floor another wing contained five men's rooms, with smaller dimensions ranging from the smallest at 3' 9" x 6' 6" to the largest at 13' 6" x 12'. A second set of stairs led to the ground floor; the plan showed a chimney; but no closets.

The second chamber floor plan shows a wing, under the eaves, reserved for the ladies. There were four rooms of various sizes: 15' x 12', 14' x 12', 12' x 10', 17' x 12' and interconnected, with one set of stairs. Separated from the ladies' rooms by a wall, and mirroring the floor below, there was another family room measuring 18' x 11', two large store rooms and stairs to the lower floors.

In April 1829 a licence application letter from Alice and Betsy Mercer stated that they intended to accommodate 25 insane persons and that such licences had been granted since 1818. Accompanying this letter was a plan for additional accommodation showing the house elevation from the front. The ground floor details three parlours, two measuring 16' x 13' 6" and one 11' x 8', a kitchen and a storeroom. Stairs led to the second floor with five bedrooms the largest at 16' x 12' and the smallest at 12' x 8', one room has a closet adjoining. Three further bedrooms were shown in the attic, with a closet; 21' x 7', 12' 6" x 7' and 19' 6" x 7'. Outside the main door to the street there was an area described as 'Front Court' onto the main street and a second 'Back' court at the rear of the building. A space to the side was shown as a garden or airing ground.

Halstock. Alice and Betsy Mercer's licence application, 1829. Its content laid out their intention to accommodate 25 insane persons and that licences had been granted since 1818. The application included a list of patients and accompanied a plan for the proposed new asylum building. DHC, Q/A/L.

List of patients at Halstock, 1829, which accompanied Alice and Betsy Mercer's licence application. The various 'classes' of patient include two members of the landed gentry, 12 are recognised by titles (women by their marital status) with the remaining seven listed, without titles, as paupers.

There is no record of the additional accommodation having been constructed and it cannot be identified on the Tithe map produced 15 years later.

None of the building records, applications, or Visitors' appraisals discuss aspects of security at Halstock. Nor was there any concern for safety regulations in relation to the patients or the neighbourhood. Security, the safeguarding of patients and public safety did not appear in any of the legislation relating to asylums throughout this period. It could be presumed that the house was locked, perhaps at all times though no comment was ever made in respect of key holders nor was the presence, or otherwise, of staff on site at all times recorded.

In 1842 the Metropolitan Commissioners reported that although the Halstock patients appeared to be 'comfortable' the property was very old and needed improvement. In the following year two of the six visits were conducted by the Commissioners. Generally their remarks tended to be more critical, focussed on the physical accommodation and on this occasion they stated that one room was found to be in a 'very filthy condition and the adjoining yard as bad'. The Commissioners also found the house ill adapted for its purpose. The upper floor sleeping rooms were within the roof space, so must be cold, and they objected to violent patients of opposite sex living so close to each other.

From 1828 the Visitors were required to turn their attention to recording detailed information about the patients and their situation as well as their accommodation. The report of October 1828, the first since the Act, began with noting the lack of a register for the medical attendant, Mr Shorland. This was with 'much regret' as Mrs Mercer had received a copy of the new regulations a fortnight previously and was considered to have had

Report made by the Visitor's following their inspection to Mrs Mercer's asylum in December 1828. The lack of a register to record their own observations was noted, although the previously requested medical register was now in place. DHC, Q/A/L.

sufficient time to act upon them. Neither was she able to produce certificates for the seven patients who were confined at the time.

Patients under restraint were now to be observed. No previous record had made any mention of restraint at Halstock asylum, but nationally this was a matter of concern. Various methods of restraint were used in asylums and workhouses across the country. Their over use was criticised by more enlightened commentators. But they were considered justifiable when preventing patients harming themselves, or others, or to stop any wandering particularly at night. It was probably used in both of these circumstances for different patients and ensured the continuation of employing few staff. Within the same report Visitors noted four males and two females, all of whom were named, placed under restraint during the day. Overnight this applied to 19 out of the 25 patients; the precise methods used at Halstock were not noted.

The report produced in October 1828 continued to record observations made which were now required under the new legislation and in particular this related to whether private patients Mr Keane and Mrs Davis should be removed. At the next visit, in the December of that year, the Visitors discovered that Mrs Davis had chosen to remain at the asylum. Mr Keane was removed in May 1829 (see his story below). The visit of April 1828 continued to record that one female remained in bed and overall the house appeared to be clean.

The accommodation of individual patients in separate areas was of interest to the Visitors and it was noted that Mr Welch and Mr Keane, both private patients, had accommodation in the newly built separate house. Importantly, and for the first time, the provision of baths was recommended along with the suggestion that 'advantages would arise from additional exercise and manual labour'. This last comment had resulted from the examination of the courtyards which were considered to be small. There was a swift and positive outcome to the Visitors' first report. A few weeks later a shower bath and a 'slipper warm bath' had been provided. In August 1830 special mention was made that the shower bath had been used throughout the Summer with beneficial, though unspecified, effects.

Without further description, it seems unlikely that the courtyards were anything more than paved areas very far from pleasant places in which to rest. It could be concluded that these spaces were reserved for the paupers and perhaps the more unmanageable private patients. However, in 1836 the Visitors instructed that a shed to be built for the female patients as a protection from the elements which implied that there was some attempt at improving the situation.

The Madhouse Act 1828 stated that 'consolation of Religion may soothe and compose the minds of patients' and participation in church services or other forms of worship was expected to be detailed in every report. Consequently, the Visitors named those thought well enough to go to church or attend any form of 'divine service'. As the years progressed prayers were read in the house generally and specifically to those who could be expected to 'derive consolation' from this particular activity. Such was the importance placed on this activity, or treatment, it was noted that for one patient, a dissenter, a Minister could have been arranged to visit the house.

The business of attracting private patients was achieved in several ways including advertising within medical journals and directories and across all areas of the medical profession.[140] Advertisements for private asylums began at least from the beginning of the 18th century and were published in journals and newspapers, also appearing in handbills, leaflets, brochures and reports. It was also crucial to highlight success rates; hence the commonly used advertising slogan 'no cure, no pay'. At Halstock it is likely that the appeal of a residence with homely standards in a pleasant area would have been the draw. For an asylum deep in rural Dorset it is probable, in the early years at least, that word was spread amongst church and court officials and those in the medical profession. Later, newspapers offered an additional method of marketing business as can be seen in an advert of 1832 where it was made clear that the proprietors were looking for 'respectable Patients':

> Halstock Lunatic asylum. There are at present TWO VACANCIES for respectable Patients in the above establishment, and persons desirous of availing themselves of this opportunity will be good enough to apply to Mesdames A. and B. Mercer as early as possible. The Surgeons are Messrs. Shorland of Yeovil. Dated Halstock, October 12, 1832.[141]

Improved documentation was now necessary to admit a patient. For private patients a medical certificate was required signed by a doctor, or other recognised medical professional, as well as a written notice from the person sending the patient. The following admission notice for a private patient, was made in 1831 by the surgeon Edward Turner:

> Mr John Haines of Yetminster Dorset has been occasionally under my care

140   Parry-Jones, *The Trade in Lunacy*, pp.102-3
141   *Sherborne and Yeovil Mercury,* 12 October 1832.

for the last four years during which period I have frequently noticed slight aberrations of his mind and this morning I found him labouring under the highest state of insanity, so much so that I consider him utterly incapable of taking care of himself and that confinement becomes indispensably necessary.[142]

The phrase 'incapable of taking care of himself' was frequently used by the medical profession in their admission notices for private patients. John Haines was moved from Halstock to Laverstock in Wiltshire, later in the same year. At the time it was known as an exemplary establishment and was said to treat its private and pauper patients with kindness and consideration.[143]

After 1828 the Visitors reports contain much more detail of the care and treatment of individual patients. In December 1828 when they recommended that the visiting doctor should attend to the 'bodily health' of Mrs Davis. Her health situation was reported during subsequent visits, she appeared to be content and 'composed', she remained at the asylum until her death in 1840.

In another new direction the inspectors also attended to the provision of improved beds and bedding. In December 1830 they stated that during the winter months patients should be provided with two 'good top blankets' and an under blanket. Earlier reports had mentioned the general cleanliness of the asylum, but the Visitors had not made specific recommendations. In October 1834 and for the first time they recommended the use of chloride of lime twice every day 'during the present heat of the weather' in the different wards and once a day at other times. This approach reflected the use of lime, amongst other chemicals, becoming recognised as a disinfectant which was thought to make an impact in reducing the transmission of diseases. The recommendation was taken up as reported in the December of that year and was not mentioned again.

The Visitors passed comment on the quality of the air in the property at almost every inspection before and after 1828. They referred to the house being in a 'wholesome state' until in March 1838 when the language changed to it being 'well ventilated, and the sleeping apartments free from any unpleasant effluvia'. The need for ventilation was primarily aimed at the removal of offensive smells in a quest to create a pleasant environment free from odours. Removal of odours almost certainly did assist in maintaining

142   DHC, Q/A/L/Private/1.

143   Parry-Jones, *English Private Asylums*, p.37.

DORSET

A Report of the House of Alice Mercer Widow and Betsy Mercer Halstock in the County of Dorset and of every Patient confined preceding the date hereof.

N° in Order of Admission	Date of Admission of Patient and by whose Authority sent	Date of Certificate of Insanity and by whom Signed	Christian and Surname Sex and age of Patient and whether Single or Married	Occupation or Profession
1	29th August 1802 by his Nephew Mr William Toogood	29th August 1802 I. Peukevill M.D. and Thomas Shorland	Robert Toogood Single Aged about 70	Yeoman
2	25th July 1803 by her Father Robert Spear	25th July 1803 Charles Hayman	Mary Spear Single Aged about 45	....
3	26th October 1807 by Edward Hawkins her Brother a Surgeon	26th October 1807 Robert Sutlock Ryme Intrinseca	Sarah Hawkins Single Aged about 50	....
4	30th June 1809 by her Sister Miss Harriet Penny of Weymouth	30th June 1809 John Daniel Beaminster	Jane Stephens Widow Aged about 70	....
5	2nd November 1809 of his own accord	2nd November 1809 I. Peukevill M.D. and Thomas Shorland	Peter Penny Single Aged about 47	Esquire
6	17th August 1813 by Lady Caroline Damer	17th August 1813 Richard Reynolds Surgeon	Jane Jefford Married Aged about 60	....
7	26 March 1814 by Mr James Mills his Brother in Law	26 March 1814 William Shorland Ilchester	James Welch Single Aged about 50	Gentleman
8	10th April 1815 by the Overseers of Frampton	10th April 1815 John Trowbridge Cerne	Thomas Barrett Married Aged about 60	Blacksmith
9	12th February 1816 by his Mother	12th February 1816 Thomas Knott Bere Regis	Joseph Sims Single Aged about 31	Gentleman

Section from Halstock's first full annual patient register, 1828-1829. DHC, Q/A/L.

SHIRE

Spinster Licenced for the Reception of Insane persons within the Parish of therein or who shall have been confined therein within Twelve Months

Parish	Whether found Lunatic by Inquisition and date	Signature of the Medical attendant and date of Visitation and observations	When Discharged	Cures Relieved or Incurable	Deaths	Signature of Visitors and date of Visitation
Motcombe Dorset	. . . .	October 25 1828 Samuel Bradley M. D.	. . . .	Incurable	. . . . .	October 25 1828 R. Gordon John White Saml Cox
Bere Regis Dorset				Incurable		
Houghton Cross Somerset	. . . . . .			Incurable	. . . . .	
Weymouth Dorset				Incurable	. . .	
Somerton Somerset	. . . .				14 May 1829	. . . . .
Abby Milton Dorset	. . . .	. . . .			24 January 1829	. . . . .
Lymington Somerset	. . . .		. . . .	Incurable		
Frampton Dorset	. . . .			Incurable	. . . .	
Langton in Purbeck Dorset	. . . .		. . . .	Incurable	. . . . .	

general cleanliness and perhaps the need for fresh air reduced incidents of illness within the property. Those reported instances of infection are few, in 1837 some patients had suffered with influenza, but all recovered and it did not spread to the whole community. In October 1840 the Visitors, having observed the physical condition and general cleanliness of the house and the patients' rooms stated that they 'do not remember to have observed them in a better state on any previous occasions'.

Aspects of the physical health of the patients in relation to their general contentment and mental health was noted occasionally from 1828 and as a more general survey in March 1838. At that time the Visitors noted that the bodily health of patients was generally good, but that one female of advanced years and '*indolent habits*' and had been indisposed. She obstinately confined herself to her bedroom and the medical Visitor recommended in '*strong terms*' her removal to the sitting room for some hours daily.

The first full annual register of patients was made in the May of 1829 (see pages 68-9). The 25 patients were listed in order of admission. Their details included: their date of admission, by whose authority they had been sent, date of certificate of insanity, by whom the certificate was signed, name, sex, age and status, occupation, their home parish, whether they had been found to be a lunatic by inquisition, signature of medical attendant, date of visitation and observations, when discharged, how discharged, the signatures of Visitors and the date of Visitation. the authority by which they had been sent was usually a church official or a family member. The methods of discharge might be cured, died, discharged to the care of relatives or relieved to another institution. The patient registers were transcribed at irregular intervals with many years missing between 1829 and 1845.

The 1828 Act had highlighted the need for Visitors to review the mental health of patients and ensure that none were improperly detained. In 1829 the Halstock Visitors considered Phillip Keane (usually recorded as of Mere, Wiltshire, but sometimes of Meare, Somerset) to be confined without good reason. He had been admitted by his wife in 1818. Ten years later the Visitors noted that he had been well for last two years and directed Mrs Mercer to write to his 'Friends' requesting his removal. It was noted that Mr Keane's friends had been due visit in a few days and that the fees for his year's board were now overdue. The Visitors stated that if he was not removed 'measures will be taken to obtain his release under the provision of the 7th Section [of the 1828 Act]'. Mr Keane had still not been removed by the following April so 'the Visitors in consequence think it is right to direct the Clerk of the Peace to take measures for bringing him to the Sessions'. The cost relating to this business was considerable, amounting to £17 16s. 0d., the details of which were described in the register's account pages. Mrs Keane, his wife, wrote to the Quarter Sessions 'praying that a representative may be made to the Visiting Justices for him to remain at the Asylum'. But the Clerk of the Quarter Sessions replied that 'steps would be taken to bring him before the Court'. He was eventually discharged in November 1829 by an Order of the Quarter Sessions and did not return to Halstock. Whether his outstanding account was settled remains a mystery, nonetheless the reference in the court records to fees, paid or otherwise, was the first recorded in Dorset. Clearly the Visitors had acted swiftly upon the new legislation relating to those who had been detained without good cause.

To prevent improper incarceration paupers could only be received with a written order signed by two Justices of the Peace or a parish overseer and a clergyman. Susan Mayo Lamb was admitted to Halstock in 1829 following a signed letter from two Justices of the Peace to the Bridport overseers of the poor.[144] She was removed shortly afterwards by the Bridport overseers in 1830, but no reason was given. Four years later in 1834 she was admitted to Forston, having been released she was admitted again in 1836 aged 34.[145]Further details suggest that the cause of her insanity was 'disappointment in matrimonial expectations', sometime violent and her mental situation said to be hereditary.

Understanding upon admittance whether patients could be cured or otherwise was not straightforward. Following an initial assessment the considered outcome was often revised after the patient had been resident for several months. Samuel Kiddle of Sydling St Nicholas was described as incurable when medical officers examined him in 1842 yet found to be curable the following year; it was unsurprising that prognosis was often altered over the years by various visiting surgeons. In contrast to the Stockland asylum, the term 'cured' was used rarely at Halstock, with only a handful of patients described as such.

The registers demonstrate that patient turnover at Halstock asylum was small and the death rate low.[146] In the year ending May 1831, when it was managing 22 patients, the register included nine private patients and seven pauper patients from Dorset with six patients from Somerset, five private and one pauper. There had been two deaths, one following a stay of six years

144 DHC, Q/A/L/Private/1.

145 DHC, NG-HH/CMR/4/32A/096 and 176

146 DHC, Q/A/L/Private/1.

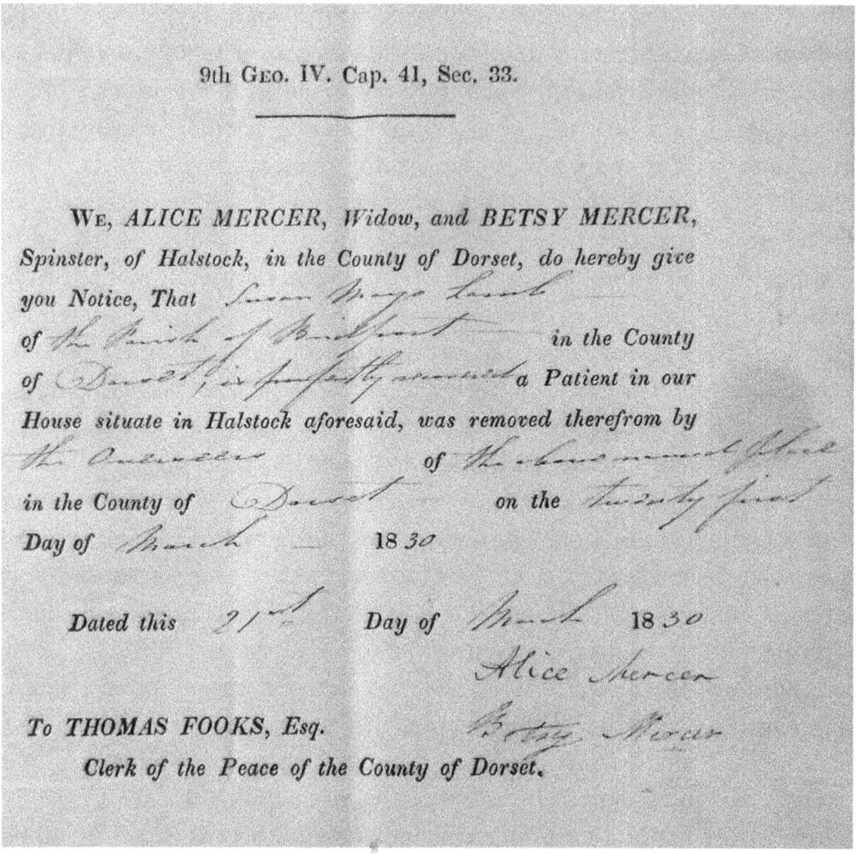

9th Geo. IV. Cap. 41, Sec. 33.

We, *ALICE MERCER, Widow, and BETSY MERCER, Spinster, of Halstock, in the County of Dorset, do hereby give you Notice, That* Susan Mayo Lamb *of* the Parish of Bridport *in the County of* Dorset, is perfectly recovered *a Patient in our House situate in Halstock aforesaid, was removed therefrom by* the Overseers *of* the above named place *in the County of* Dorset *on the* twenty first *Day of* March 1830

Dated this 21st *Day of* March 1830

Alice Mercer

To THOMAS FOOKS, Esq. Betsy Mercer

Clerk of the Peace of the County of Dorset.

Standard form used by Alice and Betsy Mercer to advise the Clerk of the Peace of the removal of a patient, here used for Susan Mayo Lamb's removal to the care of the overseers of Bridport parish, 1830. DHC, Q/A/L.

and another after a year. Two of the private patients had been confined for almost 30 years. All were said to be incurable except one, William Pearce, a pauper from Mosterton, was 'cured' and discharged after three months, but in 1834, he was admitted to Forston, aged 25.[147] In early 1831 John Haines, a private patient, who was taken after just a month to Laverstock asylum in Wiltshire, presumably at the request of his friends or family. A pauper, Thomas Barratt, who had spent 13 years in Halstock asylum, was the first to be moved, aged 74, to the newly opened county asylum at Forston in 1832. Details submitted to the court year ending May 1832 revealed of the 25 patients those deemed incurable numbered 17, two had died, one was cured, two had been relieved and in respect of the three remaining, a cure was doubtful. The patient James Hood who was 'cured' left the asylum in

147 DHC, NG-HH/CMR/4/32A/088.

November 1831 but was returned in 1842. Of the two who were 'relieved' Hannah Young left the asylum in October 1831 only to be admitted to the county asylum at Forston in January 1835. The other, a Revd Helyar was discharged in December 1831 did not return nor does he appear to have been admitted to Forston. The last three, Martha Dunford, Robert Childs, James Wellstead, who were listed as 'cure doubtful' in May left the asylum towards the end of summer 1832 and early 1833 only to be admitted to Forston in mid-1832 and early 1833. Consequently, Revd Helyar, out of 25 patients, was the only person to have 'successfully' left the asylum in that year and not returned.

When they died patients were sometimes, but not always, returned to their home parish for burial. Some were buried in Halstock without reference to the asylum whilst eight were identified in the burial registers as having been 'a patient at Mr Mercer's'. Of these John Hood, his home variously described as Netherbury and Mosterton, had been admitted to the asylum in 1831, then again in 1836. Described as 'incapable of providing for himself' he was admitted for the final time in 1842 and buried in the parish in 1847, aged 52.[148]

In 1839 after 20 years the court received an application from Alice and Betsy Mercer to 'Give up the keeping of the lunatic asylum at Halstock'.[149] The baton was now passed onto Alice Mercer's son, another surgeon, John Justinian. His application for a licence in 1838 was granted for keeping the asylum for a maximum of 25 patients for one year. The number of patients was just nine: four males and five females; no paupers were identified this time. Clearly the family continued to support each other; a letter written in 1839 from John Justinian Mercer informed John Fooks, Clerk of the Peace, that one of his patients had been moved to live with his aunt (Betsy): 'having taken Mrs Berkley under her care in the village I find by the magistrates that the within certificates are necessary'. This situation was brief and Mrs Berkely can be found returned to the asylum in a matter of months. But it highlights the flexible nature of the Mercer's care and perhaps their willingness to adapt to the individual needs of their patients.

John Justinian Mercer of Halstock was listed in the London *Evening Standard* edition of 1 February 1839 as having been granted a certificate of qualification as an apothecary the previous day. So, like his father, he was relatively young and inexperienced when he took over the asylum, although, also like his father, he had the benefit of his experienced mother and aunt to

148   DHC, PE-HAL/RE/4/1.
149   DHC, Q/S/M/1/17, f.121.

advise and assist him. Consistent with the male Mercers who served their community he swiftly found a role within the parish administration and was named as a trustee at a vestry meeting in 1838 for the construction of a school house on the field adjacent to the Church House near the church.[150] The church plot had been taken on by John Mercer in 1818 at £5 per annum and following his death in 1829 it passed to his wife Alice.[151]

By 1841 the asylum appeared to be a much reduced, yet still successful institution. In the census completed in that year the asylum was listed separately from the rest of the parish under the heading 'Public Institution Schedule'. It showed John Justinian Mercer 'resident medical attendant' aged just 25, his wife Harriett, his aunt Betsy Mercer living at 'Halstock Lunatic Asylum'. Harriett Day, aged 50, was listed as a female servant, although the census enumerator had initially described her as a patient. She probably oversaw the housekeeping details and managed the three younger servants, who were all in their early to mid twenties, Susan Way, Elizabeth Lake and Frederick Lake. Together they were responsible for the ten private patients (six male and four female) and five pauper patients (four male and 1 female) who were noted in the register for that year.

Several Halstock patients were transferred to the newly opened county asylum at Forston after 1832. Three patients were removed from Halstock to other institutions. Joseph Hunt was taken to the St Luke's, London in 1828. John Haines of Yetminster, a gentleman, was removed in 1831 to Laverstock asylum, Wiltshire, after spending a short time at Halstock having been admitted there in the same year by Miss Elizabeth Haines. Jemima West was reported in December 1836 to have been removed to Bailbrook House at Batheaston near Bath, by order of the Axbridge guardians. She had originally been admitted to Halstock, aged 41, by the overseers of Wedmore, Somerset, in March 1824, and said to be incurable. Her entry in the asylum register also noted a medical certificate dated five years earlier in March 1819 which had been issued on the order of magistrates. Her burial was recorded in the Batheaston parish register in February 1841, aged 50, her abode was given as Bailbrook House Batheaston of Axbridge Union.[152]

The following account is a request for payment made to the Wedmore parish officials in respect of Jemima West upon her removal from Halstock asylum to Bailbrook House near Bath in 1836.[153]

150   DHC, PE-HAL/CW/1/2.
151   DHC, PE-HAL/CW/1/1.
152   SHC, D/P/baton 2/1/15.
153   SHC, D/P/wed/13/2/23.

The Gentlemen of Wedmore
> To A & B Mercer Halstock
> An Acct of Jemima West

From the 12th of March 1836 to the 24th December

Thirty one weeks based at 12s. week	£24 12s. 0d.
Two weeks short of a months notice	
Previous to the Patients removal	£1 4s. 0d.
Calico & Making 7s. Flannel 4s.	£0 11s. 0d.
Gown Lining & Making	£0 9s. 0d.
Stay 5s. Worsted Hose 4s. 6d. List Shoes 4s.	£0 13s. 6d.
Shawl 5s. Bonnet 5s. 6d. Mending Clothes 5s.	<u>£0 15s. 6d.</u>
	£26 5s. 0d.

STOCKLAND

THE MADHOUSE ACT of 1828 dictated that each asylum was to receive at least four inspections a year. For Stockland, an average of three inspections were made annually by one or more justices of the peace who were accompanied consistently by the visiting surgeon Pearce Rogers Nesbitt of Honiton, who also sometimes visited alone. The Visiting Justices of the Peace were a relatively small group over the asylum's 21 year history, just seven; two were members of the church, two members of the landed gentry, and three have not been identified. Revd William Palmer, doctor of divinity and curate of Buckland St Mary, Somerset, was the Justice who made the most visits at three a year over seven years. John Hussey, a gentleman, of the Hussey family of Salisbury and later Crewkerne, visited once a year across ten years. In the last year, 1841, two new surgeons attended.

Following the Act of 1828 a more robust approach was adopted by the Visitors. Their remit was set out in the account of Thomas Fooks in May 1829 where he recorded his

> journey to Halstock and from there to Boardhays House in the parish of Stockland to take copies of the minutes of the Visiting Justices and physician, and also the list of the patients confined in both houses preparatory to making up the annual report to transmit a transcript thereof to the Secretary of State and a like transcript to Robert Browne esq. the clerk and treasurer to the Commissioners in Lunacy in London.

His journey took him away from home for three days and his fees were £3 3s. od. and there was a further cost for horse and gig hire, turnpikes and expenses of £4 19s. od.

During one of their earliest visits it was noted that patients were not receiving the required two visits a year from their 'friends', or that such visits had not been noted in the asylum journal. Spicer was instructed to improve this situation, though it was not made clear how he would do so, nevertheless by December the Visitors recorded that the patients had correctly been visited 'by their Friends' in respect of the Act.

The Visitors found Spicer had failed to keep proper records and they made it clear in March 1829 that immediate attention was required. Later in December further criticism was made in respect of an entry in the surgeon's register which described a patient as being 'not so well'. The Visitors requested a more explicit report which expressed whether this was applicable to the mind or body. The inadequate record keeping continued to antagonise the Visitors and in February 1833 they ordered Spicer to display a plan of the asylum within the property. He was also to provide a medical journal in which, as the Act required, and they specified that he was to make weekly entries.

Spicer's failure to maintain accurate records was compounded by the failures of the Visiting Justices, who rarely appeared to make much effort to record the status of the patients. This makes it difficult to identify backgrounds with any certainty. Full registers which showed by whom people had been confined exist for only four years 1828-1832 and for the last year of the asylum's operation, 1840-1841.

By 1832 Spicer was clearly wealthy and held a considerable property portfolio. He was listed as proprietor and occupier of 'Ford',–where he paid land tax of £12 5s. 11d. Spicer's property interests extended beyond Stockland he also owned and occupied lands called 'Hands Down' in the neighbouring parish of Dalwood documented in 1829 and 1831.[154] He had some status in the community as a minor local official and was named as one of the assessors for the land tax assessments in the hundred of Whitchurch Canonicorum.[155]

Through his freehold ownership of land in Stockland he was qualified to serve as a juror at the Quarter Sessions. In the jury lists he was variously described between 1828 and 1842, as a farmer, asylum master, gentleman

---

154   DHC, Q/D/E(L)/22/48/1.
155   DHC, Q/D/E(L)/59/40-45.

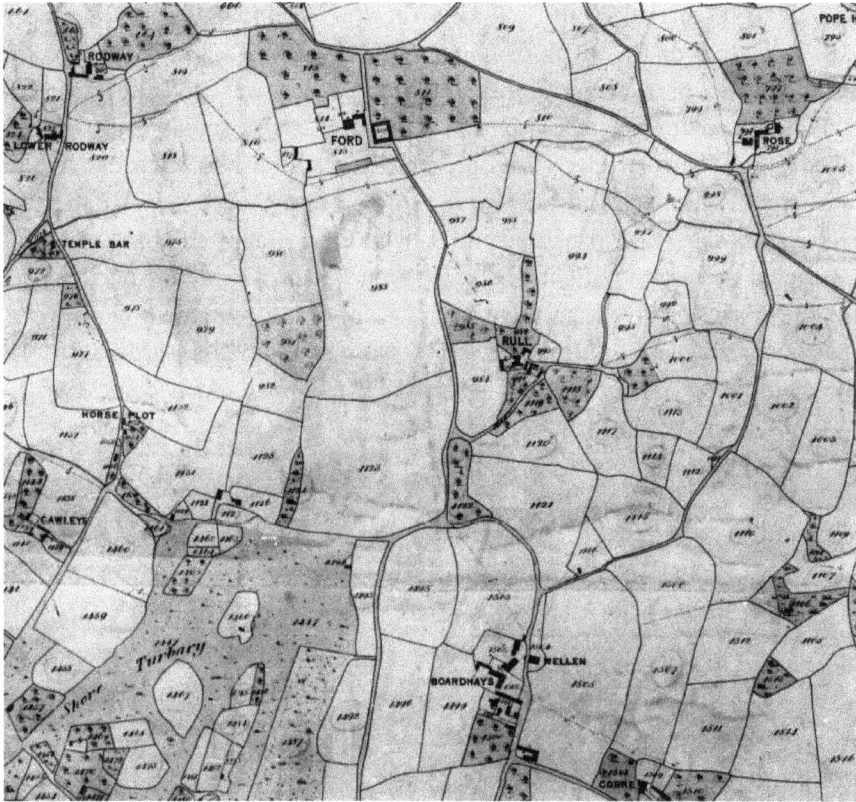

Stockland tithe map, 1844, showing Ford and Boardhayes. The accompanying apportionment named William Spicer as owner and occupier of land surrounding the Ford property identified with numbers 810, 811, 812, 813, 814, 815, 816 and 817. TNA, IR 29/10/199.

and yeoman, but never a surgeon.[156] When the tithe map was produced in 1844 Spicer's association with the asylum had reached its end although the accompanying apportionment still named him as its owner. The plot in which the asylum was situated measured over one acre, and he also held meadow, pasture and orchard lands amounting to over 56 acres.[157] His lands in Dalwood, included pasture, arable and rough grazing, as well as the house and garden occupied by the innkeeper John Anning.

The Quarter Sessions records were not concerned with noting the employees and without the existence of documents from the asylum itself the only information available is the 1841 census which showed John Davey, of Stockland aged 24, resident as the keeper of the asylum along with Ann

156   DHC, Q/S/J/5/1842/34.

157   TNA, IR 29/10/199.

Genge, aged 19, and Sarah Daw, aged 18, who were both domestic servants.

Several of the areas of concern remained the same as before the introduction of the Act, continued importance was given to whether the areas under inspection were 'free from offensive smells' and whether the rooms were properly ventilated. The provision of natural airflow was frequently observed and in 1828 a recommendation was made that ventilators should be 'procured and used in the passages' and used in rooms occupied by certain patients. Following a number of epidemic occurrences in the early 19th century there was a recognition that the environment, particularly where a number of people were living in close proximity, was likely to present a risk.[158] Clearly this knowledge had reached some of the

Report of the Visitors on conditions at Stockland made in March 1829 by William Tucker and Francis Goforth, the Justices of the Peace assigned to inspect the asylum. They record that the ventilators requested were now fitted and two patients, Samuel Dean and Joseph Huxter were under restraint. Apart from some failure in keeping a required record it appears that they found the rest of the house in good order. DHC, Q/A/L.

158   Tempel, Wouters, Descamps and Aerts *Ventilation techniques in the 19th century,* p.271.

court officials and they were keen to advise that mechanical means were now available to assist with the removal of foul air, replacing it with fresh air. A few months later in March 1829, the Visitors reported that ventilators had been fitted.[159]

A shocking discovery was made in the March of 1837 where the Visitors found 'a small sleeping room used by a helpless female requires immediately to be repaired'; this room can be seen in the plan of 1830. They continued to report that glass and 'apertures' to be mended to prevent 'free access' to rats. They also found a sitting room used by male patients filled with smoke from 'foulness of chimney' and requested that it should be swept immediately.

A plan of the Stockland asylum dated 1830 was submitted to the Dorset Quarter Sessions. This is probably the document that accompanied Spicer's original application for a licence in accordance with the Madhouse Act of 1828 repurposed to demonstrate the division of male and female patients as required by the Quarter Sessions.

A plan, dated 1830 and identified as 'Boardhays', was annotated and signed by Spicer. It contains little description relating to the rooms and their functions, providing only a simple layout over two floors in the 'north wing' with a basic drawing of a separate three storey building with cellar. The plan offers few further details, simply noting the 'Entrance hall', above that a 'bedroom floor' and finally a 'garrett floor'. Spicer added that 'there are two rooms in two of the airing grounds where the patients go to warm themselves which are not drawn on this scale'. He further stated that Boardhayes was to contain no more than 20 licenced lunatics. The outside space is not shown on this plan and no further plans for this date exist. Following the requirements of the recent 1828 Act this effort was unlikely to impress the magistrates responsible for granting Spicer's licence, it has none of the detail shown on the drawings created for Halstock asylum in 1828.

A second drawing, which is undated and unnamed, includes a list under the heading 'In the New Buildings'. It sets out the ground floor rooms and 'Chamber Story', all numbered with details of their purpose, differentiating male and female occupation. The drawing is self explanatory, but worth noting are two bedrooms, one above the other (4 & 14), both measuring 36' x 17' which were expected to house ten female patients in each. There were two Day Rooms for female patients, one on each floor, measuring 18' x 17' (nos 2 & 13) with a space noted as 'Ward robe' on the second floor (no.12). The male sleeping areas covered three rooms. The

159   DHC, Q/A/L/Private/1.

Plan of Stockland asylum at Boardhayes House, 1830, showing all floors of the property. William Spicer noted his intention to accommodate a maximum of 20 lunatics. DHC, Q/A/L.

largest of these was 30' x 17' with a corresponding bedroom above each for nine patients (nos 5 & 15). The additional smaller bedroom measuring 14' x 17' was to sleep four male patients (no 16). The two male day rooms were on the ground floor; one included a bath. A matching bath room for female patients is not shown.

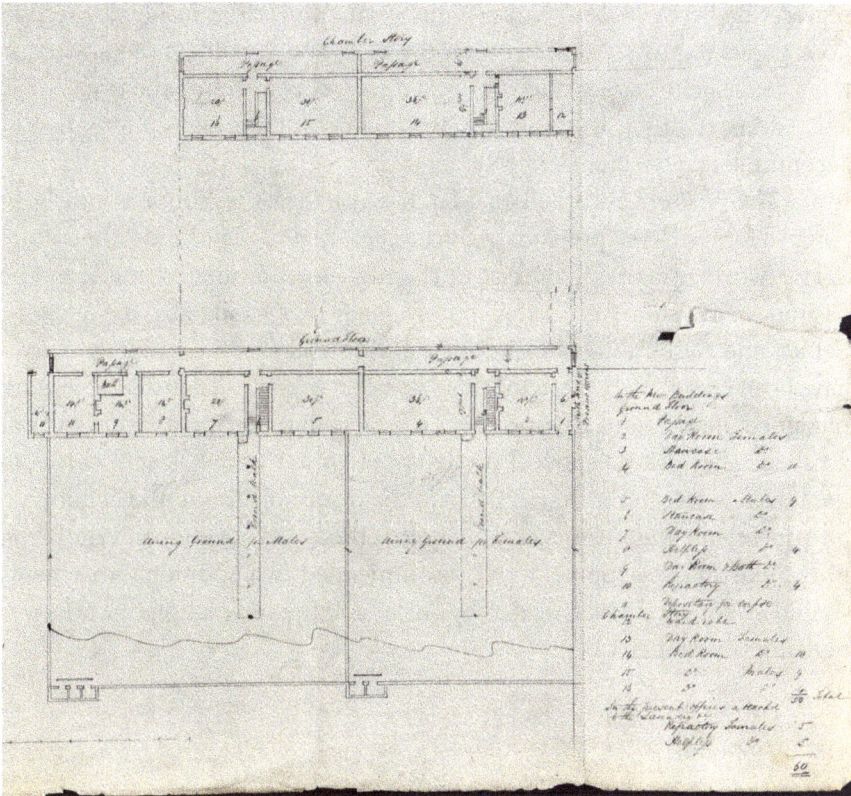

Plan of Stockland asylum (perhaps unbuilt), undated, and at an unknown site. The plan gives details of each room with its purpose and the number of patients expected to occupy the space. The importance of segregating the sexes is recognised and expressed on the plan. The building was to accommodate 60 patients.
DHC, Q/A/L.

A further two rooms were designated for the 'Helpless', one of which is drawn on the plan and shows accommodation for four males on the ground floor (no.8) and measured 14' x 17'. The female 'helpless' room, for five patients, is not shown but was described as near to the offices and laundry. Another room is labelled with the term Refractory and was designated for four unmanageable male patients situated on the ground floor 14' x 17' (no 10). The similar Refractory room for five female patients is again not shown but said to be beside the laundry. The small room on the ground floor numbered 11 was named as the depository for corpses.

Movement around the building was facilitated by separate staircases for men and women between floors and doors leading to the outside area known as the Airing Grounds by means of a 'covered walk'. Here the segregation between the male and female patients is clear. Inside, the second floor passage shows a wall between the male and female quarters whereas the passage below appears to suggest a doorway connecting the two.

Importantly it was noted on this plan that there was an intention to accommodate 60 patients.

The Visitors recorded in March 1834 that 'the house is nearly in complete repair' yet previous reports neglected to determine the nature of this work, a marked contrast to the high level of interest taken by the Visitors at Halstock. A further report made in October by the Visitors, Palmer and Nesbitt, stated that despite agreements that the buildings should have been completed by August this was not the case and considerable work remained outstanding. By April 1835 the 'sleeping apartments' were still not finished. The Visitors showed particular attention to the sleeping areas of the house where in the winter of 1830 the inspectors found the bedding to be insufficient. The Visitors also noted that there was not enough ventilation in the existing development and recommended two additional casements should be added; this was agreed by Spicer and the completion of works was noted in September 1835.

A regular Visitor's report made in 1839. The report describes the escape of a patient; the walls built as a result of the escape and the insufficient clothing supplied to the pauper patients. DHC, Q/A/L.

The property appears to have been extremely secure. Remarkably few escapes were made or made known to the Visitors. The three escapes which were reported reveal something of the nature of the buildings and the efforts that had been put in place to secure confinement. The first instance was reported in February 1839, a male patient had twice escaped over the walls of the court, the outside space where patients took exercise. At the time of the report the walls were said to be in the process of being build up to a height of 14' all around the property. The second escape was in October when two pauper patients succeeded in 'wrenching an iron bar from one of the windows which had been but imperfectly riveted'. Now repaired the Visitors noted that the property was fully secured and despite initially eluding capture the two escapees had been returned.

After William Spicer had given up the asylum another interested party, John White, submitted a licence application in June 1843 to continue the asylum at the Ford House site.

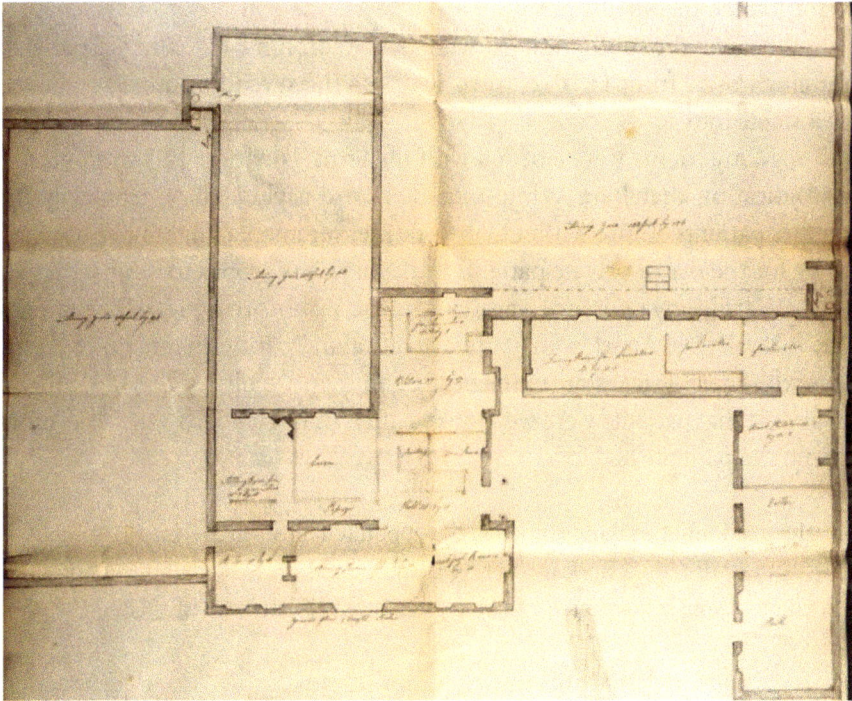

Stockland asylum, located at Ford House, showing extensive layout of rooms designated for the 'lunatics'. The plan accompanied John White's application to the court for a licence in 1843. DHC, Q/A/L.

The plan of the ground floor of the principal building shows a hall, 20' x 10' store room, pantry and kitchen at 20' 6" x 17'. The kitchen led to a sitting room, 14' 6" x 10' said to be for lunatics. Returning to the hallway passage the plan shows a larder and another slightly larger sitting room, again for lunatics, measuring 15' 9" x 15'. Three further rooms are described as a parlour at 15' x 11', a large dining room 24' 6" x 14' and breakfast room 15' x 14'. A door from the parlour leads to one airing ground measuring 111' x 93'.

Upstairs there were two additional bedrooms for lunatics one measuring 13' 6" x 18' 6" and the other 16' x 13' with three further bedrooms, a dressing room with bedroom and a drawing room. No provision for one or more baths is shown.

The outbuildings show a stable, coach house, cellar, and back kitchen measuring 18' 6" x 17' 6", which was linked to two rooms designated for 'lunatics' patients, without dimensions, and another linked to their dining room, at 27' x 13' 4". A doorway led out to the airing ground measuring 132' x 106' which included a privy.

Above the outbuildings were six bedrooms for lunatic patients ranging in size from 11' x 10' to 19' x 17' 6". The seventh room was labelled as a stable loft.

Many rooms were labelled with the term 'Lunatics'. This was perhaps an indication that John White intended Ford asylum to be primarily for pauper patients. Those without labels or measurements might have been set aside for the use of private patients or the asylum's proprietor and staff.

Hardly any reference was made by the Visitors relating to the patient's day to day living. Apart from matters of diet and security, their main concern, was with the physical state of the house and they usually expressed a general overview that patients were well looked after. In December 1828 the Visitors found the patients had

> the freedom of walking abroad at the appointed hours in the yards assigned for their use', they 'appear to be well and humanely treated and the house commodiously fitted up for the purpose for which it was used.

It appeared that most, if not all, the inmates had some interaction with the Visitors where possible, as noted in June 1829, where one was 'now conversing freely' and another more 'composed' and better. It was regarded as of great importance, and always reported, that there should be an availability of religious observance on Sundays. It was apparent in Stockland, prayers were not being held regularly on Sundays.

The visiting surgeon, Pearce Nesbitt, was certainly concerned with the welfare of the patients, often recording comparatively lengthy (when compared to the other two Dorset asylums) reports to the court. In December 1830, he noted that two patients needed every attention as 'their bodily health' was very unsatisfactory. He advised that a daily record should be kept containing details of the 'symptoms, treatment and termination of every malady'. He continued to show a level of knowledge and progressive thinking as can be seen in August 1831 when he recommended that Hannah Thomas, who had been confined in the asylum for nine years, be discharged on trial. He said that she had been 'labouring under occasional mental derangement' of severe epileptic paroxysms which are irregular periods leading to ordinary epilepsy. He considered her to be otherwise rational and thought a 'trial ought fairly to be given to her removal from hence with a view of ascertaining whether her present malady may not be benefitted by the change'. Hannah was discharged and did not return to Stockland.

The Visitors rarely made a distinction between the treatment of paper and private patients but, in March 1838, they noted that the pauper lunatics were 'very badly clad' and said that they did not know how to 'meet this evil'. Spicer assured them that he would follow this up with the 'respective parochial authorities' who were responsible for providing clothing in addition to their regular weekly maintenance charges. Two months later it was reported that some of the patients 'seem better clad'.

In a new departure, and one which was not explored at Halstock, was the attention paid to the food provided to pauper patients. In April 1837, due to 'circumstances having occurred' the Visitors reported that the meals given to the paupers should be investigated. It seems that though the 'dietary scale of the Axminster Union has been acted upon' they were concerned with the quantity and quality of the food stating that it was not 'sufficient for lunatics whose bodily health is good'. The Axminster Poor Law Union diet, supplied in the workhouse at Axminster, is set out in Appendix 3. Also supplied in the Appendix is a copy of the diets supplied at Forston and at Hanwell asylum, Middlesex. Hanwell was regarded as a model institution and the advantages of the institution's diet were highlighted by Sir William Ellis in his pioneering *Treatise on the Nature, Symptoms, Causes and Treatment of Insanity*.[160]

The discussion moved on a few months later when, in September 1837, mention was made of Hanwell County Asylum (Middlesex) which suggest that the Visitors were aware of some practices outside the area. Hanwell was the model presented in Ellis' 1838 treatise which made various general and specific recommendations relating to improvement of institutions

160   Ellis, *A Treatise on the Nature, Symptoms, Causes and Treatment of Insanity.*

across the country. Hanwell's approach to patient care was progressive and alongside gentle employment it was believed that a nutritious diet aided recovery and was particularly beneficial to pauper patients. Evidently the Dorset Visitors were aware of Hanwell's novel approaches to patient care before the publication of Ellis' influential report the following year as in September 1837 the Stockland's keeper was 'cordially disposed' to follow the Hanwell diet.

However, despite efforts made by the Visitors it was reported six months later, in March 1838, that the change of diet had 'disagreed with the patients and that at present no regular system in this respect seems to be acted upon'. The subject was considered again in November 1839 when the Visitors 'interrogated some of the more intelligent patients separately with the view of ascertaining if they were properly taken care of' which seemed once again, due to complaints received, to be diet related. However, during the same visit it was witnessed that the dinner appeared to be 'a sufficient meal with which they were satisfied'.

Although William Clarke Spicer had received his licence in 1820 the first entry in the Quarter Session records recording the conditions of the patients at Stockland did not appear until December 1828. At that time the Visitors recorded nine men and five women of whom two men and one woman had been restrained by some means due to violence 'lately exhibited'.

Patient numbers rose through the 1820s to reach 22 by 1830, over the next three years they fell to 15 in 1833 before rising again to a peak of 29 when the asylum closed in 1841. Throughout the period in which the asylum operated paupers outnumbered private patients, perhaps by as many as five to one if those unclassified patients were all paupers (see Appendix 1). Men always outnumbered women, the usual ratio being around two to one. Although in the later years many patients were not classified as private or pauper, it appears that paupers usually outnumbered private patients by at least two to one.

There was a high turnover of patients with frequent admissions, removals and re-admissions. Overall, the asylum had admitted over 100 known patients across its comparably short existence of just 21 years, at an average of 4.7 per annum.

In May 1830 there were 23 paupers in residence most of whom had been confined during the previous year. One, Peter Tolman, had been removed on trial, four had been cured, two had died, eight were thought to be incurable and eight were considered curable. A majority, 13 paupers, were from Devon, with seven from Somerset and three from Dorset, they had all been admitted by their parish overseers. Four of the seven women and eleven men were married and whose occupations included butcher, labourer, shoemaker, waggoner, mason, cooper, yeoman, and gardener. The register showed that the certificate of insanity prior to admittance was often signed by a Northcote Spicer of Chard, surgeon and brother of the asylum proprietor William Clarke.

For the same period there were six private patients, four male and two female. Of these five were said to be incurable and one curable, William Wheadon. William, aged 27, had first been admitted to Stockland in December 1828 by his mother from his home in Seaton, in Devon, his occupation was given as chemist and druggist. The records show he was removed by his sister in October 1829. But by March 1830 his name appeared once again in the Visitors' report though had been he was removed on trial. He was readmitted just two months later, now incurable and again removed on trial in January 1831. William had made a will in 1828 which was proved following his death in 1831, in which he left everything to his mother, Mary.[161]

Samuel Dean, was listed at the outset in 1820, described as a yeoman, aged 50 and single from Chardstock in Dorset. He had been admitted by his brother and remained at the asylum until his death in 1837. The Visitors reports recorded that he was often under mechanical restraint during his confinement across 17 years. Another private patient, Joan England, was unmarried and aged 54 when she was first listed on the court register. From South Petherton, Somerset, she had been admitted by her sister in 1820 and spent the last 13 years of her life in the asylum.

For pauper patients entry to the asylum was negotiated by either the patient's family, the overseers of the poor in the parish, the poor law union and workhouse board of guardians or a combination of these interested parties. One such patient, William Clarke, was admitted to the asylum in 1838. A settlement examination in respect of his widow Hannah took place the following year in 1839 which gave more information about the family and their situation. William Clarke's wife and family had lived in Southleigh for 31 years and during his last illness they had received relief from the Honiton Union until William was put into the asylum at Stockland by the overseers of Southleigh, he was said to be 'out of his senses' and died soon after in October 1838.[162]

The pauper patients were usually from one of the nearby poor law unions and tended to remain at Stockland for the duration of their treatment.

161   TNA, PROB 11/1788.

162   DvnHC, 3327 A/PO 82/62.

DORSET

A Report of the House of William Spicer Licenced for the Reception of every Patient confined therein or who shall have been confined therein within

Nº in order of admission	Date of Admission of Patient and by whose Authority Sent	Date of Certificate of Insanity and by whom Signed	Christian & Surname Sex and Age of Patient and whether Single or Married	Occupation or Profession
1	February 21. 1820, by her Sister	February 21 1820 Northcote Spicer Chard	Joan England Single Aged 54	
2	February 25 1820 by his Brother	February 21 1820 Northcote Spicer Chard	Samuel Dean Single 50	Yeoman
3	April 1st 1822 Wm Johnson Esq	April 5th 1822 Northcote Spicer Chard	James Baldwin Single Aged 38	Gentleman
4	May 7. 1822 by John Perris her Husband	May 7. 1822 Northcote Spicer Chard	Elizabeth Perris Married Aged 45	
5	November 8th 1822 by the Overseers of Axminster	November 8th 1822 Samuel Symes Axminster	Mary Farrant Married Aged 46	
6	February 9. 1823 by the Overseers of Honiton	February 19. 1823 J. C. Serrard Honiton	Hannah Thomas Single Aged 39	
7	June 10. 1825 by the Overseers of Banwell	June 10. 1825 Thomas Austen Gols-brough	Barrow Harvey Married Aged 45	Yeoman
8	October 17. 1825 by the Overseers of Chard	October 17. 1825 Samuel Wear Chard	Thomas Hayball Single Aged 39	Laborer
9	June 24 1826 by the Overseers of Axminster	June 25 1826 Northcote Spicer Chard	William Cross Single Aged 62	Shoemaker
10	August 11. 1826 by the Overseers of Axminster	August 9 1826 Charles Hayman Axminster	Joel Bowren Married Aged 60	Laborer

Section from Stockland asylum patient register for 1830-1831 as transcribed for the Quarter Sessions. The list names both private and pauper patients who were all said to be incurable. DHC, Q/A/L.

SHIRE

Insane persons within the Parish of Stockland in the said County of Dorset and if Twelve Months preceding the date hereof 30 May 1831.

Parish	Whether found Lunatic by Inquisition and date	Signature of the Medical attendant and date of Visitation and Observations	When Discharged	Cured Relieved or Incurable	Deaths	Signature of Visitors and date of Visitation
S. Petherton Somerset	. . . . .	1830 June 16 Pearce R Nesbitt M.D	. . . . . .	Incurable		1830 June 16 Wm Tucker Fred Goforth
Chardstock Dorset	. . . . .		. . . . . .	Incurable	. . . . .	
Barnstaple Devon	. . . . .		. . . . . .	Incurable		
Colyton Devon	. . . . .		. . . . .	Incurable	. . . . .	
Axminster Devon	. . . .		. . . . .	Incurable	. . . . .	
Honiton Devon	. . . . .		. . . . .	Incurable	. . . . .	
Banwell Somerset	. . . . .		. . . . .	Incurable	. . . . .	
Chard Somerset	. . . .		. . . . .	Incurable	. . . . . .	
Axminster Devon	. . . . .			Incurable	. . . . .	
Axminster Devon	. . . . .			Incurable	. . . . .	

However, one, Barrow Harvey, a yeoman admitted in 1825 from Banwell in Somerset, aged 45 was removed, on an application from the overseers of Banwell parish, to Ridgeway House in Stapleton, Gloucester in 1832. This was a small establishment licenced to surgeon Dr Nehemiah Duck which, in the census of 1841, suggested it admitted private patients. In the same census 1841 a Barrow Harvey was listed, now aged 50 and living at Bailbrook Lunatic Asylum in Bath, Somerset, which was a larger establishment housing both private and pauper patients; the document noted that he was born in the county.[163] He died in 1846.

Paupers who were considered to be idiots, rather than lunatics, were incurable and likely to be removed to accommodation within the parish or poor law union. Mary Perry arrived at Stockland in February 1833 and described as an idiot a year later by the Visitors. As a result she was to 'to be given up' to the overseers at Axmouth 'when a proper habitation shall be provided in which there are no young persons'.

In contrast to Halstock asylum, a high number of patients were removed from Stockland 'on trial' and were returned to their communities to assess their current status and ability to remain at large. The visiting doctor, Pearce Nesbitt, was proactive in trial releases which had been part of the legislation made in 1828. Dr Nesbitt appeared to be more aware than most contemporaries of its potential advantages to the paupers who made up the majority of Stockland's patients or, a less charitable view, perhaps he was under pressure to release people back to their parishes. Yet, for the fortunate ones, the term trial release appears to have been applied not only to those who were considered to have been cured and were deemed sane, but also to those who were thought to have been confined without reason.

The June of 1830 saw the release of patients who were certified and endorsed as cured by the newly appointed Dr Nesbitt: Hannah Emmett, John Hamlett and William Wills. Another, James Harding, was also to be discharged 'as soon as the overseers of Musbury shall certify that security has been given that he shall be chargeable to the parish of Musbury to which he belongs'. They had all left the asylum by September though William Wills was readmitted in February 1833, he was not cured and was admitted to Forston in 1842.

Cure rates appear to be quite high in number and were keenly recorded but only after due process had been observed by the Visitors - three visits with 21 days between each. Across the lifetime of the asylum patients released now 'cured' amounted to 28, with only four of these

Report of August 1831 stating Hannah Thomas and Henry Rowe are to be discharged, the latter now said to be sane. Visitors, Francis Goforth and John Hussey, note that Burrough Harvey and Henry Hammett have not received the required regulatory visits. The report demonstrates the difficulties found in assessing suitability for discharge. DHC, Q/A/L.

were later admitted to Forston. The apparent willingness to discharge patients at this rate could be thought at first commendable, but as their eventual outcome was not evaluated it could be presumed that many returned to a cheaper option for the parish which was likely to have been the workhouse. On the outside it looked good for business as a high cure rate was mentioned by asylums in their advertising. Perhaps the regular visiting surgeon felt conditions at the asylum, for some at least, were unsuitable and although they had not been cured they would fair better in a different environment.

In respect of prompt payments of fees Stockland, which accommodated a large number of pauper patients, probably did not suffer from the same levels of default that may have afflicted those asylums that specialised in private patients. Nevertheless, there were disputes relating to the place of settlement of the patients and therefore which parish should pay for their care. In October 1835 the Visitors reported a patient named Wilkins, said to be a dangerous idiot, had been placed at the asylum by a Devon magistrate's order. His occupation and settlement could not be ascertained. A year later in 1836 his case was discussed at the Dorset Quarter Sessions where it was confirmed that his place of settlement was the parish of Saint Cuthbert near Wells in Somerset.[164] The overseers of the poor from Saint Cuthbert appealed unsuccessfully against a fee chargeable to them of £37 7s. The sum included the initial removal and 14s. per week charged by Stockland asylum for maintenance, medicine and clothing. In March 1837 the Quarter Sessions recorded an application from the overseers at St Cuthbert's Wells for Wilkins to be discharged to the parish workhouse. The removal order was duly signed to discharge 'the said idiot on payment of all reasonable charges'. The 1841 census lists a John Wilkins in the Wells Union Workhouse, Priory Road, aged 40, he was still there 20 years later when the 1861 census gave his place of birth as Glastonbury.[165]

Some people were considered to have been confined without reason, such was the situation for George Major, a labourer from Netherbury who was admitted in July 1831. Dr Nesbitt felt that he did not present 'mental derangement' and called for a further investigation. By December of that year Major's sanity was agreed by both the Visitors and Spicer and his discharge was subsequently ordered. His brother, Samuel Major, had also been a patient at Stockland admitted by the overseers of Netherbury in May 1830, aged 24, a labourer and said to be 'curable'. He was recommended for discharge in the December of the same year. Curiously, a George Major from Netherbury was admitted to Halstock, aged 27 in July 1840, and released, said to be cured the following March. A George Major, aged 35, from Netherbury, was admitted to Forston in 1837, said to be suffering from hereditary insanity.[166]

Another patient, Samuel Crabb, was seen by Dr Nesbitt in June 1831 when he was assessed to be 'so well as to be entitled to his discharge'. In February 1840 Mr Palmer and Dr Nesbitt made a special visit to the asylum

164   DHC, Q/S/M/1/17, f.16.
165   Census, 1841 and 1861.
166   DHC, NG-HH/CMR/4/32A/218.

Stockland patient list, 1839. DHC, Q/A/L.

to determine whether two paupers should be released. It was decided Robert Clapp should be freely discharged with no conditions attached and that Elizabeth Applin should also be released 'on trial' and subject to recall. These actions may have been the best outcome for some, for others they clearly did not provide a long term solution. They certainly demonstrate genuine concern on the part of the Visitors and that some periodic reassessment took place. It was clear that focus on the rights and wrongs of confinement was avoiding the basic need to raise the standards of care, which were rarely mentioned, or to look for better methods of treatment.

The Visitors report of November 1839 focussed on concern that there was no proper 'classification of the different inmates, paupers and boarders being indiscriminately thrown together' and private patients now being referred to as 'boarders'. They directed that this should be rectified immediately. Six months later the Visitors found the problem unchanged despite constant recommendations on their part. The difficulties continued, in April 1840 they were unable to see the male patients as they had been locked up together. Both the manager and keeper were absent. The Visitors were clearly concerned with this oversight, as well as their personal inconvenience, and ordered that it was imperative 'a keeper should always be on the spot'.

The Visitors, Revd William Palmer J.P. and Dr Pearce Nesbit, reported in April 1840 the absence of the Stockland asylum's Keeper and Manager. They could not see the male patients nor had the proper classification of patients been resolved. These problems contributed to the demise of Spicer's asylum.

By January and February 1841 the writing was on the wall for Spicer's asylum. The court officials reported that repairs remained undone and that the patients had still not been classified. They were also unhappy about the cleanliness and clothing of the patients; a hope was expressed that the asylum would be closed immediately. The general dissatisfaction with the conditions at the asylum and Spicer's failure to comply with their recommendations can be clearly seen in one of the last reports made by the Visitors in February 1841:

We have visited the asylum at Ford this day, and have seen the patients and find them nearly in the same state as they were at our last visit (Jan 25). All the patients directed to be discharged at our last visit are gone with the exception of Robert Morey who is still retained but from what cause we cannot understand in consequence of the absence of Mr Spicer, we lament that neither the window nor the house have undergone the least reparation since we were last here and again order that it may be immediately attended to, and also the classification of the patients, which we are much surprised should have been so long neglected, although our orders have been repeatedly given. We are also dissatisfied with the state of the Clothing as well as the want of cleanliness in the whole of the patients. We also suggest the propriety of each of the bed rooms having the number painted on the door - the communication between the men's yard and the adjoining one still remains open but we hope it will be closed immediately in consequence of the escape of two patients since our last visit but who have been returned to the asylum, We beg further to remark that an order was given for its being closed on Oct 29 1839.[167]

The same Visitors returned one month later, in April, which showed perhaps the level of concern for the conditions and management. They found that the 'helpless female', named as Elizabeth Turner, had been removed by the Bridgewater guardians to the workhouse within the previous few weeks.

In 1841 the census, which was taken in June, listed eleven men and seven women confined in Stockland at the Ford Asylum a short time before its closure:[168]

William Stuckey, aged 50, whose origin was not stated (and perhaps unknown).
James Baldwin, aged 50, from Barnstaple.
Isaac Ironside, aged 45, from Lyme [Regis].
Archibald Thomas, whose age was not known, from *Loaders* (probably Loders).
James Mitchell, aged, 60, from Ottery St Mary.
John French, aged 92, from Kilmington.
William Wills, aged 80, from Beer.
Benjamin Wyatt, aged 22, from Upottery.
William Cross, aged 78, from Axminster.
Henry Hammett, aged 52, from Barnstaple.
Osmond Baker, aged 41, from Pinhoe, by Exeter.
Elizabeth Perris, aged 53, whose origin was not stated.
Henry Ford, aged 53, whose origin was not stated.
Diana Hart, aged 31 from Sidmouth.
Martha German, aged about 40, whose origin was not stated.
Ann Bond, aged 53, whose origin was not stated.
Mary Farrant, aged 59, from Axminster.
Maria Symonds, aged 30, from Ilminster.

A letter from Spicer in July 1841 to William Fooks, clerk of the peace, accompanied a copy of the list of 'inmates' at Ford House which seemed to express a sense frustration or desperation. He wrote:

167   DHC, Q/A/L/Private/1.
168   Census, 1841.

'I beg you will excuse its being done in great haste you accuse me of neglect in not making my returns regularly I beg to say I <u>have done</u> <u>so</u> immediately on the admission, removal and death of all the patients to the Metropolitan Office in Lunacy by order of the clerk there.'[169]

The final entry for the asylum appeared in the Quarter Session records in August 1841 though at the time the fate of Spicer's asylum would have probably been unknown to him. The Visitor's Palmer, Coles, Hussey and surgeon Holland reported that the patients seemed tolerably healthy and the 'statement relative to the dietary, we consider to be very satisfactory.' All orders formerly given by the Visitors appeared to have been carried out, rather too late it seems. Spicer had also informed them that Dr Selway of London had visited under the direction of the Court of Chancery and that he had expressed his 'abbrobation (approval) of the management of the Lunatics'. The reason behind the attendance at Stockland asylum was most likely in respect of the patient James Baldwin.[170] As a ward of court James Baldwin, of Ford near Stanton [Churchstanton], in Devon was the subject of such a visit in March 1840 to ascertain his current state of mind. From as early as the Middle Ages people such as James Baldwin, a landowner and judged to be a lunatic, were protected in law and by the benevolent guardianship of the monarch.[171] The court was ultimately responsible for the administration of his estate and the maintenance of both himself and family.[172]

Spicer continued and applied for a licence as usual in October 1841, it was initially moved to renew by Robert Gordon and seconded by Revd James Templer, though granted for a four month period only. The recorded entry proceeded with George Loftus who stated that the licence should 'not be renewed' a motion which was then seconded by Henry Frampton. The licence was revoked by a decisive 18 'ayes' 5 'noes'.[173] No explanation for this decision was recorded in the minutes, but Spicer's years of failure to comply with the recommendations of the Visitors must not have gone unnoticed. The official licence, which had already been drawn up, for the asylum to continue for 13 months was dated and sealed 19 October 1841. But it was later annotated in pencil 'licence refused by the justices in session'.

169   DHC, Q/A/L/Private/3.

170   TNA C 211/4/B341.

171   Lands of the Lunaticks Act, 1324, c.12.

172   Rogers, *In the Course of Time*, p.11.

173   DHC, Q/S/M/1/17, f.205.

Stockland's final report made by the Visitors in August 1841 noted that the diet as now supplied was very satisfactory and that all 'Orders' which had been previously requested had now been dealt with. The Court of Chancery's representative, Dr Selway, had visited and made known his approval of the establishment. Attention was made once again to religious activities brought to the patients who could not attend church by either the manager or his daughter. DHC, Q/A/L.

Six months later at the Quarter Sessions in January 1842 it was noted that the asylum was no longer licenced and the visiting magistrates were instructed to ensure it was not illegally open.[174] The situation was reported in the newspaper at some length which included the detail that 'the proprietor praying for an extension of the licence for a limited period, as he was in treaty with Dr Neville, for the purchase by the latter of the asylum'. But in the unanimous opinion of the Justices they could not renew the licence to the current proprietor even though the asylum 'might be eminently desirable and necessary'. As a result Spicer, in January 1842, informed the Axminster Union of the closure:

Mr Spicer, Master of the Ford Lunatic Asylum gave notice to the board, that in consequence of his asylum being no longer licenced, the paupers of the union in his establishment must be shortly removed. When the clerk was

174   Ibid., f.215.

requested to apply to the master of the Forston Asylum near Dorchester to ascertain if they could be received into that establishment.[175]

In April 1842 it was suspected that the asylum was still operating, illegally; the justices were empowered to investigate and report their findings to the court and begin legal proceedings if required.[176] By October 1842 it was reported that as there was only one patient in the asylum it was no longer under the jurisdiction of the justices.[177] The details of the removal of patients and the whereabouts of Spicer were not recorded, although parish records show that by June 1842, he had married a Malana Harris in Bristol.[178] Spicer died six years later, his burial recorded in Stockland in 1848, he was 62.[179] Three years later his widow Malana Spicer can be found on the census of 1851 living in Kilmington, Devon, with boarder James Baldwin aged 60, an ex-patient from the asylum, and probably the single patient who remained resident at Stockland when the asylum closed. Baldwin continued to board with Malana until his death in 1878. As a ward of the Court of Chancery, the administration of his personal estate was granted to the solicitor for the affairs of H. M. Treasury, his estate was worth just under £3,000.[180] William Spicer's estate was left to Malana. His executors were Thomas Deane of Chardstock and James Wakely, his son-in-law, both described as gentlemen.[181]

The fate of the eighteen patients was largely unrecorded. Some can be traced via the 1851 census which showed two private patients returned to their families (Isaac Loveridge and James Mitchell). Two male pauper patients went to Forston asylum and three were eventually admitted to the Devon county asylum at Exminster, a village on the outskirts of Exeter, which opened in 1845.

For a short period interest in the asylum continued and this interest came from John White, a farmer and not from the county according to the 1841 census. It is difficult to understand why he wished to take on the business; he must have known about the property and all the problems associated with running an asylum through previous dealings with Spicer.

175   TNA, MH 12/2096/253.
176   DHC, Q/S/M/1/17, f.223.
177   Ibid., f.242.
178   Bristol Archives, P/St MR/R/3/11.
179   DvnHC,1215A/PR/1/13).
180   National Probate Calendar (Index of Wills & Administrations) 1858 - 1995
181   TNA, PROB 11/2101/389.

Perhaps there was encouragement to do so from parish officials or the poor law union, the opening of the Devon and Somerset county asylums were still a few years away. But both were in the early stages of planning so it must have been evident that pauper patients would soon be accommodated elsewhere. Forston was full by 1841, few patients having been admitted from Stockland; so pressure for places in the vicinity remained high in the short term.

It appears that John White did not have expertise in the area of lunacy nor was he a medical man. Records available showed him as a yeoman and owner occupier of several plots of agricultural land in Stockland.[182] Nevertheless on the 10th of June 1843 John White wrote from Ford House to J Fooks (clerk of the peace) of his intention to apply for a licence. He said that Mr Holland would be the attending 'medical gentleman'. Later in the same month two justices of the peace, Coles and Palmer, wrote a letter of support to the Revd Harry Farr Yeatman, chairman of the Quarter Sessions. They said that it was the opinion of the Visitors that John White and his wife were competent to keep the lunatic asylum lately licenced to Spicer at Ford in Stockland and 'we consider under all circumstances that the appointment would be proper'. In response to White's application the court decided against granting him a licence because of a non-compliance of Section 20 of the Lunatic Asylums Act, 1842, where a statement was required regarding whether both male and female patients were to be received and, if this was the case, numbers of each sex were to be given and means of separation explained.[183]

On 29th September 1843 White wrote again, this time with the required details of patient classification. His application for a licence at the next sitting of the Quarter Sessions at Dorchester was 'for the reception of insane persons, that I intend to reside therein and that the said house and premises are capable of containing 20 male and 12 female patients'. He continued to state that the patients would be kept 'distinct and apart from each other' according to the plan of the house and premises.[184]

Shortly afterwards in October 1843 John White informed Fooks, clerk of the peace, of his decision to delay his licence application until the next Quarter Sessions because Ford House was in a 'most dilapidated state'. It was never re-submitted. A few years later John White, of Stockland appeared in the Sun (London) newspaper in March 1849 in a list of Insolvent Petitioners.

182   TNA, IR/29/10/199.

183   DHC, Q/S/M/1/17, f.275.

184   DHC, Q/A/L/Private/1.

He was shown on the 1851 census living with his wife and two daughters at Goren Villa, Stockland.

CRANBORNE

C RANBORNE WAS 'AN ancient market town in a fine open country', the largest parish in the county, and 'a place of high antiquity, famous in the Saxon and Norman times for its monastery, chase, and lords'.[185] The majority of its inhabitants were farmers or connected with agriculture in some way. Cranborne Manor, seat of the marquess of Salisbury, was placed at the heart of the village and was a significant local employer. The family seat of Lord Ashley, later the 7th Earl of Shaftesbury and a significant figure involved in the reform of asylums, was at Wimborne St Giles approximately two miles away.

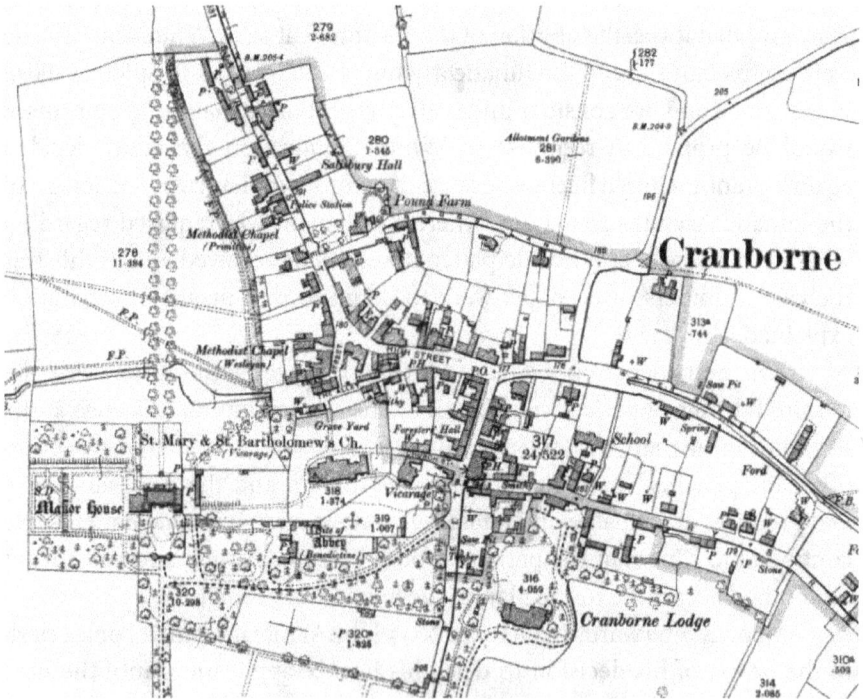

Cranborne, Ordnance Survey map 1903.

Cranborne asylum opened after the 1828 Lunacy Act had come into force. From the start it was overseen by the Quarter Sessions and had regular

185   Hutchins, *History of Dorset*, III, p.375.

visits who reported on the conditions they found. It was opened in 1830 by William Symes, then aged 43, for private patients only. William was born to parents Thomas and Hannah in Great Wishford, Wiltshire, where he was baptised on 15 August 1787.[186] It appears he did not marry, nor did he have a family living in Cranborne or nearby. His earliest connection to the village seems to be his apprenticeship to Robert Smart, surgeon at Cranborne, in 1801.[187] There was a history of surgeons being resident in Cranborne dating back through the 18th century. In 1731 Matthew West, surgeon, had leased a burgage plot called the Copped Hall within the town, and in 1795 James King, who was a surgeon resident in Cranborne, leased several properties in Woodlands from the Shaftesbury estate.[188]

William Symes rented a house in Cranborne from at least 1818 and gradually increased his holdings to include both residential and agricultural property. The land tax assessment register showed him occupying unspecified property owned by the marquess of Salisbury 1818 -1819.[189] He remained at the same property ten years later in 1828 when it was assessed to make an increased payment.[190] By 1831 Symes was renting a house, used as the asylum, from Mrs Miles at £1 16s. 3d. The same year he and a Mr Harvey, were renting a barn and plot for 5s. from James Williams,[191] which were possibly the plots of land opposite the asylum referred to in the 1840 tithe apportionment as occupied by Symes. The land tax records for 1832 noted a penny increase in the assessments for both properties. Unlike the Mercers at Halstock there is no evidence of Symes' further activity in the parish. He did not, for instance, serve as a churchwarden or an overseer of the poor.

In 1830 Robert Smart and William Symes were listed as the two surgeons listed in Pigot's Directory for Cranborne.[192] William Symes, esq. remained listed as one of the two surgeons in Cranborne in 1848, the other being at this time Edward Hill.[193] The landowner from whom Symes rented his land was Charlotte Miles, widow of William of Wimborne St Giles. It

186 WSHC, 1160/3.
187 TNA, IR1/70.
188 Shaftesbury estate archive, LE/43 and 872.
189 DHC, Q/D/E(L)/17/1-21.
190 Ibid.
191 Ibid.
192 *Pigot's Directory*, 1830.
193 *Kelly's Directory*, 1848.

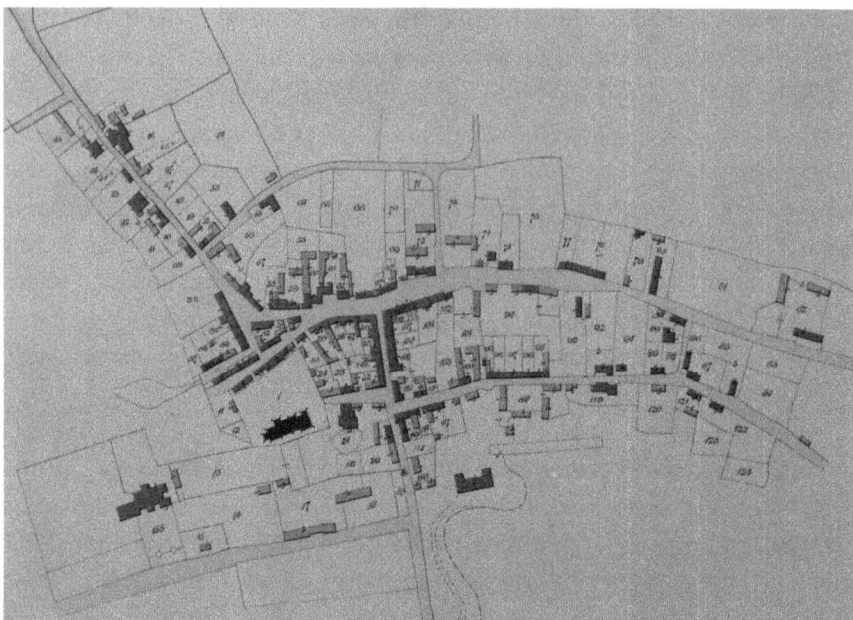

*Section from the Cranborne tithe map, 1840, The asylum 'House, Garden &
Buildings' were located at number 42 (top left). Further properties rented by William
Symes are presented including Penny's farm (number 82); gardens and buildings
(numbers 47, 47a, 48 & 49, opposite the asylum). He also farmed land in the area
under the ownership of Charlotte Miles. DHC, T/CRA.*

was Charlotte Miles who owned the asylum property, the house, garden and
buildings, which was leased to Symes along with a garden and buildings
opposite and across the road from the house. Further property nearby
was leased by Symes, a coach house and garden, from the trustees of the
Stillingfleet Charity and two gardens from James Williams also situated
opposite the house.[194]

The property, which was to become the asylum was located on Main
Street (later renamed Salisbury Street) on one of the central roads running
through the village, it is now a Grade II listed building.[195] There is no
indication that it was purpose built as an asylum, although William Symes
was one of the property's earliest occupiers, perhaps even the first. It was a
modern and impressive building in a prestigious location.

When Symes announced his intention to run a lunatic asylum
in the heart of the town there were objections from various members of

194   DHC, T/CRA.

195   National Heritage List for England, Manor View, 31 Salisbury Street,
No.1304241 (accessed 12/11/2024).

the local community. In 1830 a letter of protest was written by Colonel Frederick Griffiths to the Home Office with a plan of the intended lunatic asylum building.[196] His objection was principally focused on the asylum's close proximity to neighbouring households. Griffiths' letter of objection was signed by some eminent local people including Richard Brouncker of Boveridge, Mrs Monro of Edmonsham House, Revd Robins, rector of Edmonsham and Mr R. Smart of Cranborne. This last was perhaps the same Robert Smart to whom Symes had been apprenticed. Additional objectors were the asylum's immediate neighbour Mrs Skinner and Frederick Griffiths himself, on behalf of his sister Mrs Stillingfleet, another neighbour.

Clearly, some of Symes' immediate neighbours had raised the support of some very powerful voices in the local community to campaign against the creation of the asylum. Those who had opposed the establishment of the institution were owner/occupiers of substantial properties close in the near vicinity. In addition, the Stillingfleet family leased the coach house and part of garden opposite the proposed asylum house to Symes as the Trustees of Stillingfleet's Charity.

The letter stated that the complainants believed that a lunatic asylum would be an intolerable nuisance and

> that it is impossible for any keeper to be answerable for the continuance of a lucid interval of the patients during their walks and therefore a source of alarm to all persons who may encounter them in the fields and lanes, especially females and children.

Ultimately the petition and local objections were unsuccessful largely because the Home Department had no legal authority to intervene. Symes was able to go ahead with his plans, was granted his licence and the asylum was opened in the same year. The records do not show how Symes and his asylum were eventually received by his neighbours; there were no reports either in the court records or newspapers of the type of incidents which the people of Cranborne feared. Patients gradually became known to the town's population through Sunday church services and would have been encountered around the village.

Despite objections William Symes was granted a licence for his 'private madhouse' in October 1830 for no more than three patients which, considering that the property could potentially house many more, perhaps was an attempt by the court to mitigate local concerns and objections. The

196 TNA, HO 52/7/119, ff.271-6.

Quarter Sessions record showed he had been looking after one insane person, Frederick Dale, since 1827.[197] Maintaining a single resident lunatic did not require a licence and was a regular and expected way of supplementing income for those in the medical profession. Colonel Griffiths gave an indication of this state of affairs when he said in his letter that the asylum 'is moreover unnecessary and uncalled for there being two or three in the vicinity superintended by medical persons of the highest character, and reputation'. Griffiths provided no additional details, but his reference was probably to the town's two other surgeons, Robert Smart and Edward Hill, who may each have managed a single private patient without the need for a licence.

In 1830 only two privately funded patients were in residence in William Symes' asylum. Numbers of patients varied little over the 18 years during which the asylum operated. Mostly there were five rising occasionally to seven and in the final year there were eight patients, four men and four women. Presumably at some time the Quarter Sessions awarded a licence for more than three although no increased licence has been located. In contrast to Halstock and Stockland all the patients were privately funded; there were no paupers.

Over the years at least 20 private patients passed through the asylum, 16 were listed in the Quarter Session registers and the remainder have been identified from admission documents. One patient who did not appear in the asylum's registers or in the UK Lunacy register was a Mr Brown who was removed by 'friends' in November 1848 and taken to Bedlam by Symes. The majority, twelve patients, were from Dorset, two from Wiltshire and four from elsewhere Cambridge, Brighton, two from Jersey and two of unknown origin.

Cure rates are difficult to establish. From the Quarter Session records and UK Lunacy registers there appears to be just one cured, with two relieved, one of whom, Jane Lanning was admitted to the asylum at Fisherton, Wiltshire, in 1856 and one was discharged incurable.[198] One was removed and sent to the workhouse, two recovered and two died. Five followed William Symes to his next venture, an asylum at Grove Place, Hampshire, another went to Westbrook House, a private asylum in Alton, Hampshire; there is no information relating to the fate of the other four.

197   DHC, Q/S/M/1/16, f.156.

198   WSHC, A1/560/3, Register of Admissions, with minutes of visitors, 1813-1868.

Occupations recorded for the 12 male patients admitted to Cranborne asylum included a mechanic, hotel keeper, army captain, medical man, clergyman, yeoman and innkeeper, four were married and six were single, their average age was 47. Of the eight women three were married and five were single; with their average being 40. One female was just 13 years old.

The asylum appears to have been a contented house with a homely atmosphere. Perhaps Mr Symes was in a position to make a reasonable judgement about who would 'fit' best in a house of so few patients in which he was also resident. The Visitors reported on a number of occasions they found the 'family were at dinner', the food described as 'good and abundant' and the house appears to be 'conducted very much in the manner of a private family'. They regularly recorded the good health and kind treatment.

Church attendance was a regular activity for the patients from the asylum's beginnings. As the years progressed very few additional past-times or activities were introduced even though by this time these were understood to be good therapy. The Visitors noted that the patients were usually reading or in the kitchen. The 'very good' gardens attached to the property offered opportunities to take 'sufficient out door exercise'. It was also recorded that the patients made daily visits to Mr Symes' farm and that they 'enjoy much liberty'.

William Symes appeared to make a genuine effort to assist in the recovery of his charges and treated them more as lodgers than patients. A level of freedom was remarked upon in June 1843 when the Visitors found Mr Ferris away with his brother in Weymouth and William Symes accompanying the two Blandford sisters to Abbotts Ann near Andover, a distance of 30 miles. The Visitors also noted in 1844 that the Revd John Carnegie, a local clergyman, made visits to the house and 'engaged with Mr Almond in religious conversation'.

The house and ground plan of 1830 includes a note which must have had some importance.[199]It showed the situation of the house with access to the open fields at the rear of the garden 'in the field adjoining this door is a footpath leading to the country without passing through any part of the town'. Perhaps this alluded to the objections that had been made by local residents and highlighted in an effort by Symes to come to some accommodation with them.

The Entrance Hall, door leads to the Withdrawing Room, 16' 5" x 16' 5". The hall leads to inner hall with staircase up or down or both (note - under staircase to a cellar under the parlour and of the same size). Another door leads to the pantry, no sizes are given. The back door leads to garden.

199   DHC, Q/A/L/Private/2

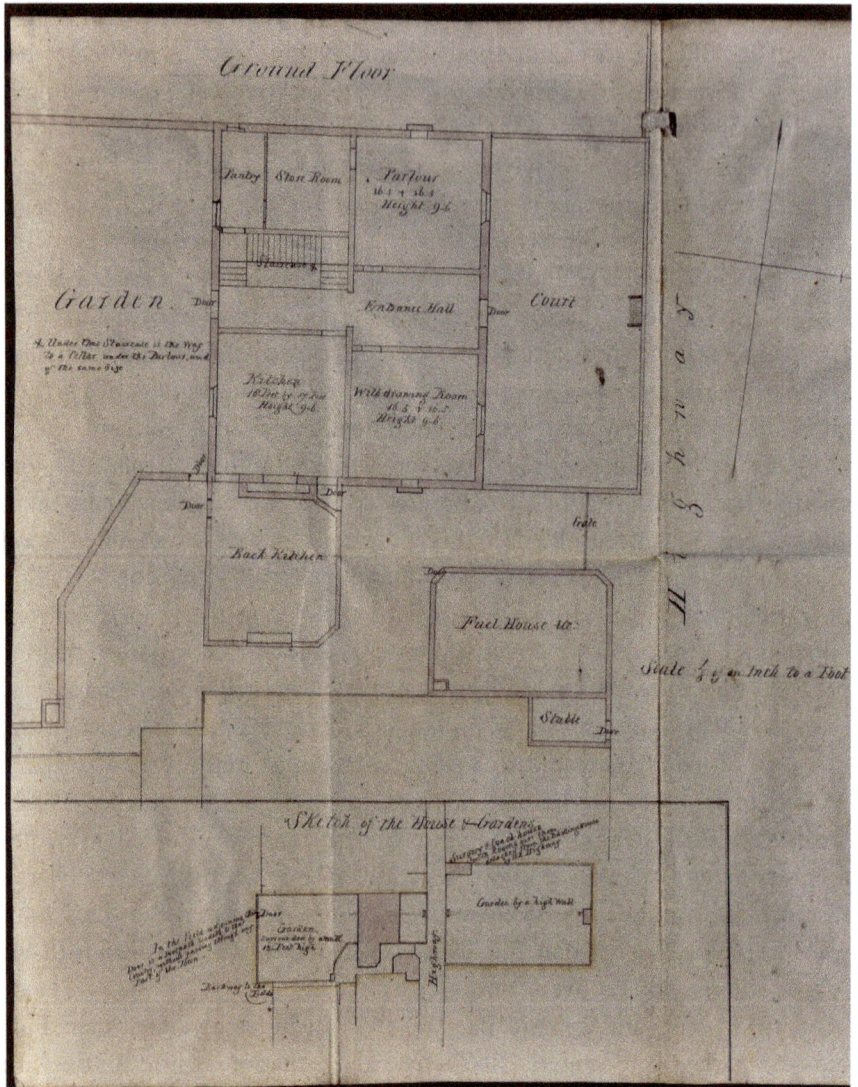

Cranborne plans of the asylum, 1830. 1. (above) showing ground floor and location of the house and gardens, 2.(opp.) showing the first floor and attic rooms. DHC, Q/A/L.

Access into the kitchen 18' x 17' is from the main hall. Opposite there is a parlour, the same size as the withdrawing room, with a door to store room, no sizes. Another door, possibly from the outside access to area with 'Gate' leads to the back kitchen. A door from this room leads to an outside passageway to 'backway to the fields'. Across a path there is a fuel house etc and stable. The garden at the rear of the house has a wall of 12' surrounding it with the door, as mentioned above, leading to the fields beyond.'

First Floor

Chamber
16 Feet by 11.6

Chamber
16.5 + 16.5
Height 9.6

Staircase

Landing

Dressing Room
11.6 + 9 feet

Closets

Chamber generally
used as a Sitting Room
18 by 17 Feet Height 9.6

Chamber
16.5 + 16.5
Height 9.6

Chamber over
Back Kitchen

Landing

Highway

Scale ⅛ of an Inch to a Foot.

Attic

Door
10 by 12.6

Door

Staircase

Landing

19 by 14 Feet

19 by 16 Feet

19 by 16 Feet

Immediately opposite the front gate of the house and across the highway, there is a garden 'by a high wall'. In the corner by the road there is a building described as a surgery and coach house with rooms over them detached from the dwelling house by the highway.

Upstairs, there are 5 bedrooms, chambers. 16' x 11' 6"; two 16' 5" x 16' 5" above the withdrawing room and parlour, one said to be generally used as a sitting room 18' x 17'. with 2 closets. There is a dressing room 11' 6" x 9' above the front door and hall.

The 5th bedroom is over the back kitchen which offers no dimensions so it could be presumed this was for staff or Symes himself.

Stairs rise to the attics where there are four rooms, presumably bedrooms; three are identical measured at 19' x 10', with the fourth room smaller at 10' x 12' 6". There is no indication of a bathroom or provision of bathing facilities, but these may have been included in the room furniture, though not included in the list of items for sale in the 1849 auction.

The drawings appear to show three main bedrooms with another, used at the time as a sitting room, which could have been brought into use as a fourth bedroom. The attic floor had three sizeable rooms which were used for patients, two sisters shared a bedroom throughout their stay, and a smaller room perhaps used for live in staff. Therefore, the resulting bedroom space appears to make for comfortable accommodation for six to possibly eight people. It seems from the records that this maximum number of people boarding in the house occurred only for a short time in 1844. Despite frequent requests Symes was restricted, under the terms of his licence, to a maximum of five patients only.

Symes employed a number of staff including, according to the 1841 census, at least four who were resident in the asylum. All were 20 years old: Anna Green was described as the housekeeper, while Mary Joy, Eliza Joy and Thomas Edwards, were all described as servants and were probably recruited locally as all had been born in Dorset. At that time there were six patients, so including Symes, the surgeon and keeper, the staff to patient ratio was five to six. Three years later, in an extensive Visitor's report compiled by Moss King, Thomas Edwards, was described as a competent 'indoor' servant who was able as part of his duties to assist with the management of the patients. A few weeks later another Visitor, Henry Sturt, reported that Edwards was in charge of the male patients and that he 'never leaves the house in case of the absence of Mr Symes'.

Some brief biographical details of the residents accommodated at Cranborne are illustrative of the mix of private patients under William Symes' care. The youngest by far of all the Dorset asylum patients was Elizabeth Nation, aged just 13 when she was admitted to Cranborne asylum on 21 March 1847 by Amelia Webber. The admission record described Amelia Webber as a governess from Blandford, so presumably she had been appointed to look after Elizabeth prior to her admission. The admission notice stated that she was an idiot from birth, the medical examiners said she was 'incapable of giving a rational answer on any subject a state of fatuity (stupidity)'.[200]

Elizabeth's origins are obscure, but she may have been born to Maria Nation in February 1834 in Walcot St Swithin, Somerset, where a Maria was listed in the 1841 census, aged 35, with a female servant. Maria's likely burial place was Bath Union workhouse graveyard in December 1849, aged 43. The same census of 1841 showed Elizabeth Nation, aged 5, living at Mount Pleasant, Walcot, which may have been some form of institution as the other inhabitants were two women and three men, all with different surnames. There was no further information recorded within the records for Cranborne about where she was placed when the asylum closed. A girl by the same name was listed in 1851 census in the Bath Union workhouse, aged 16, and she may have been the Elizabeth Nation buried in 1874 at Bedminster St John, Bristol, at 38 years old. Elizabeth was not recorded at Cranborne as being a pauper. Someone had paid for her maintenance and treatment at Cranborne, and someone had employed her governess, Amelia, at Blandford, but their name was not provided in the admission papers or by the Quarter Sessions.

Jane Oakley, a married woman from Blandford aged 45, was first admitted in October 1840 by her brother-in-law Angel Symes, a hatter by trade. After two years, in November 1842, she was discharged from asylum, considered cured. A month later, in December 1842, the Visitors found a woman in the house who was 'restored to her reason' and said to be the assistant housekeeper, the Visitors also noted that she had a 'distant connection' to William Symes though no familial relationship with him was stated. On examination the Visitors reported that she gave 'some good reasons' to remain and that she appeared 'perfectly rational'. No name was mentioned but by March 1844 the Visitors noted that Jane Oakely had been appointed six months earlier, in October 1843 to the role of housekeeper and superintendent of the female patients, a salaried position, during the occasions William Symes was away from the asylum.

However, soon afterwards in June the Visitors reported that Jane Oakley had once again been officially confined to the asylum as a patient which was confirmed in the register of 1844-1845. She was officially admitted by her brother-in-law and guardian, no details of her condition or likelihood of cure were given.

In May 1845 she was the subject of discussion when it was noted that she had not benefitted from a visit made by the vicar 'whose attention was specifically called to her by Mr Symes'. In the same report the Visitors recommended that iron bars should be placed in her room though, unusually, Mr Symes took exception to this suggestion as he 'thinks it would be objectionable in the present state of that patients health'. There was no further comment on the matter.

In one of Cranborne's last reports of September 1848 the Visitors said that they found a female patient suffering with 'melancholy'; possibly referring to Jane Oakley. After the asylum closed she went with William Symes to his new venture, the Grove Place asylum in Nursling, Hampshire.[201] Then, in June 1855, when William Symes had left Nursling, she was admitted to Fisherton Anger asylum, Wiltshire, where she died in 1863.[202] Her estate with 'effects under £800', was granted to her sister Sarah Hodges and husband Angel.[203]In life she was said to have suffered from an 'everlasting misery'.[204] which would be considered in current times likely to be clinical depression.

James Almond was known to be residing at the asylum in 1841, the census showed him to be aged 20 and from 'foreign parts', having been born abroad. When he was first seen at Cranborne by the Commissioners in Lunacy they found that, although he had been a resident of the past four years, he was not strictly a patient; no certificate having been provided. It was declared that he was under treatment for epilepsy and continued to live at the asylum without the necessity of admission paperwork nor was he under any inspection from the Visitors. This was an unusual outcome as at the time epilepsy was a condition which continued to be regarded as a form of insanity and treated as such. The register showed he was eventually officially admitted in January 1844 by his mother and remained there until moving to Grove Asylum at Nursling in 1849, along with the other patients from Cranborne. He was listed in the 1851 census, at Grove, which was annotated with the note 'lunatics age and where born unknown'. In 1855 he can be found listed in the Fisherton Anger asylum register, aged 37, where

201   TNA, MH 94/8, Oakley, Piece 08.

202   WSHC, A1/560/3, Register of Admissions, with minutes of Visitors, 1813-1868.

203   National Probate Calendar, (1863, Oakley) 1858-1995.

204   DHC, Q/A/L/Private/3.

he had been admitted from Grove Place, his trade said to be a linen draper.[205]
He was discharged '*not improved*' in October 1868 and next appeared in
the census of 1871, a patient at the Jersey lunatic asylum where he had been
baptised in St Helier in 1817, he was now 54. Eight years later his burial was
recorded in 1878, aged 60 in St Helier with the cause given as 'softening of
the brain'.[206]

Two long term Cranborne residents, the sisters Mary Ann and
Charlotte Blandford, were born in Fifield Bavant, Wiltshire, a small parish
about 10 miles north of Cranborne, to parents Thomas and Ann in 1799
and 1803.[207] The sisters lived in a large farmhouse with their seven siblings
until they were admitted by their brother, also Thomas, to the asylum at
Fisherton. Mary Ann was admitted in October 1828 and Charlotte in
September 1832. Their medical certificates were signed by another brother,
George. Both sisters were removed in November 1836, not cured, and placed
in Cranborne asylum the same month. Much of their time passed with little
comment apart from a report in June 1843 which noted their excursion to
Abbots Ann, a distance of some 30 miles, accompanied by Symes. A few
months later it was noted that one of the sisters did not attend church.

Census records show that the sisters remained in asylum care
throughout their lives; moving from Cranborne first to Grove Place,
Nursling, with William Symes and then to Bagatelle Retreat in Jersey
where they resided with Isaac Pothecary in 1861.[208] In 1871 Mary Ann and
Charlotte were recorded as 'Lodgers', still with Isaac Pothecary, by which
time the asylum was known as Cranborne House.[209] The census of 1881
shows the sisters living with their niece, Mansel Blandford, 39, in Braganza
House in St Peter's parish, Jersey, all three described as living from 'income
from interests of money', with a cook and a housemaid.[210] The enumerator
noted their condition as 'imbecile'. Mary Ann and Charlotte remained with
Mansel until their deaths a few years later, buried within weeks of each other
in January 1885. They were said to be aged 81 and 77 though their baptism
records would suggest that they were older.[211] Their estates combined

---

205 WSHC, A1/560/3, Register of Admissions, with minutes of Visitors, 1813-
     1868.

206 Jersey Archive, G/C/03/A4/9/2.

207 WSHC, 1052/9.

208 Census 1861, Jersey.

209 Census 1871, Jersey.

210 Census 1881, Jersey.

211 Jersey Archive, G/C/03/A4/9/2.

amounted to over £4,000 which was granted to Mansel, their next of kin.[212] Mary Ann had spent 57 years in care and Charlotte, 53.

James Foss was the only patient who was said to have been 'cured' during his stay at the asylum. He spent three months at Cranborne between December 1830 and March 1841. He was the innkeeper of the Black Bear in Blandford Forum, tenant to owner John Bragg. His name was recorded on the jury lists for Blandford Forum from 1825 to 1830 and 1835 to 1837. His death in September 1837, aged 49, was published in the local newspapers.[213] It seems likely that the families who sought to place their relatives in William Symes' care had already come to the conclusion that they were unlikely to be cured and that they should be afforded a tolerably comfortable life.

A licence was granted in 1830 for 'keeping a house for the reception of insane patients at Cranborne' for no more than three patients and, in line with legislation of 1828, local magistrates were required to inspect the asylum, at least four times a year. The following year the numbers of patients were not specified. The Justices appointed for this task were Henry Sturt, Revd Moss King and Hector Bower Monro, with John Rowe of Wimborne the visiting surgeon.[214] John Rowe appeared to have been most diligent in his role often visiting alone to make assessments and attend to concerns. This can be seen in August 1843 when he made a special visit to meet with James Almond, finding him to be of sound mind. Rowe was not adverse to making recommendations independent of the justices of the peace and during the same visit he requested a small alteration of two windows.

There were 18 inspections made between 1830 and 1841. However, none of these visits were made or reported to the court for six years from 1833 to 1838. Nor, during this time, were records of fees or licence payments made in the accounts section of the Quarter Sessions court register. Although there were no formal visits during this period it appears from private correspondence that John Rowe, the surgeon, visited the asylum in September 1833 and December 1834. Otherwise the asylum was visited by those justices appointed at the original grant of the licence with the additional appointment of Richard Brouncker.

The first recorded visit was made in December 1830 by the Justices of the Peace Moss King and Henry Sturt. They found that there were two patients and recorded their satisfaction with the establishment. Over the next two years there was no change, numbers remained the same and the

212   National Probate Calendar (Index of Wills and Administrations 1858-1995).
213   DHC, PE-BF/RE/4/1.
214   DHC, Q/S/M/1/16, f 199.

inspectors were satisfied with their conditions. The reports were mostly short and concentrated on the state of the house and cleanliness of the patients; all criteria were met. The only exception was in August 1831 when there was a recommendation that the windows of bedrooms occupied by three patients should be secured by iron bars to prevent a patient throwing himself out of the window. Symes took his time over this instruction and the bars were not in place until December.

Henry Sturt visited Cranborne in his capacity as one of the official asylum Visitors. His report, made in November 1839, included the usual details of the house with an additional focus on church activities mentioning a patient who had disrupted a Sunday church service. DHC, Q/A/L.

By the late 1830s the attendance of church services was under scrutiny, again a result of the 1828 Madhouse Act. In November 1839 the Visiting Justice Mr Sturt, reported that one of the patients, Mr Dale, was unable to go to church, having been banished by the vicar for interrupting the service. In line with the Madhouse Act, those who were unable to attend church received prayers at the house together with the sermon, all of which had to be recorded and reported to the visiting inspectors. This was a matter of on-going concern for the Visitors who in 1840 reported that one of the patients who had occasionally attended the church now appeared 'attentive to his duties and attends the church regularly twice on a Sunday'. Aside from church attendance the earliest mention of any kind of activity at Cranborne, was in April 1840 when the Visitors recorded that the two female patients and two male patients had been gardening and out walking.

William Symes was often reported as being absent when inspections took place. It was a matter of concern for the Visitors and was regularly highlighted in records made to the court particularly after 1840.

The court documents demonstrate that Symes frequently failed to comply with the necessary legislation or pay much attention, it seems, to directives from the Visitors. Possibly his difficulties stemmed from a lack of understanding, a generous view perhaps, but either way the situation was not helped by his failure to bind up a copy of the 1828 Madhouse Act to the inspectors book. This task remained undone more than a year after it had been requested in July 1841 when he was also asked to display the required plan of the house.

The Visitors made few references to Symes' record keeping, perhaps he complied adequately with the requirements regarding the medical condition of the patients, admissions, removals and deaths. Lapses in providing the correct paperwork was possibly overlooked or even sidelined because the Visitors found little fault with the overall care of the patients and generally the comments reflected that the asylum was well conducted in every respect. However, although the keeping of accurate records was not, it seemed, a major concern, the keeping of a lunatic without a licence was less easily overlooked. In October 1841, this situation brought about a motion in the Quarter Session that William Symes be prosecuted for keeping a lunatic, James Almond, without a licence.[215] Yet a few months later, in January 1842, he was granted a licence without further comment.[216]

There is a small amount of correspondence among the Quarter Sessions records relating to the Cranborne asylum which gives an insight into the character of William Symes and his suitability to manage the institution. The first is a letter to the clerk of the peace, Mr Fooks, in October 1838, in advance of the Michaelmas Quarter Sessions, which provides direct evidence of his involvement with the daily treatment of his patients. In it he states:

> I should be very glad to have a renewal of a licence for my house for the reception of insane patients and as you request me I will if possible be at Dorchester tomorrow morning by the Mail [coach], but I have some patients at this time who require my daily attendance...[217]

215   DHC, Q/S/M/1/17, f. 205.
216   Ibid., f. 214.
217   DHC, Q/A/L/Private/3.

An endorsement for Symes and his asylum came from a high level at the Michaelmas Session of 1838, when the Earl of Shaftesbury wrote the following observation on a copy of the licence: 'I consider Mr William Symes of Cranborne to be a proper person to have a renewal of his licence for keeping a house there for the reception of insane persons.' Shaftesbury was one of the leading protagonists involved in legislation relating to asylums and this cannot have passed unnoticed by the Quarter Sessions. He is unlikely to have given Symes his approval with some knowledge of his character, perhaps as a visiting surgeon at Wimborne St Giles for his estate workers or even his own family. However, it was another five years before Shaftesbury would visit the asylum at Cranborne in an official capacity.

The following year, in 1839, William Symes wrote to Mr Fooks, stating his intended attendance at the Michaelmas Court Sessions, but explained that in the event he had been unable to leave home. The letter appealed to Mr Fooks in the 'hope you will procure the licence for me', sending £10 in part for licence, and he continued to say a cheque would follow to cover what was due. He continued 'if the magistrates will give leave for me to have six patients it would be of great service to me, I have plenty of rooms for double that number'. His request was probably borne out of a realisation that the asylum needed more patients in order to survive.

That William Symes managed to keep the asylum as long as he did showed some tenacity. It also showed a certain lack of any real power from the court with whom he had been at odds on many occasions. The first problem occurred in October 1839 when he was granted a licence for only four months rather than the usual term of a year.[218] This was direct evidence of an institution in special measures, but no specific reason was given for the short period of renewal.

Two years later in 1841 the court recorded a notice that at the next Sessions the Clerk of the Peace should be instructed to prosecute Symes for keeping a lunatic asylum without a licence.[219] The situation was made public in the newspaper. Robert Gordon, Justice of the Peace, pointed out that the licence had not been renewed and though there were no charges of mismanagement the 1828 Asylums Act required a licence, which brought the asylum within the jurisdiction of the magistrates and by not doing so 'Mr Symes was saving 15s. a year which ought to go to the funds of the county'. Notice was given to proceed to indict Symes for this failure.[220]

218 DHC, Q/S/M/1/17, f.138.

219 DHC, Q/S/M/1/17, f. 205.

220 *Salisbury and Winchester Journal*, 25 October 1841.

A letter from Edward Du Bois, Clerk and Treasurer to the Metropolitan Council in Lunacy, was received by Mr Fooks, Clerk of the Peace in Dorset in October 1841, which said that Symes had not been providing returns in accordance with 1834 Poor Law Act 'the neglect of which places him in some danger'. Du Bois continued to explain that he needed copies of orders and certificates with admissions of all the patients who were resident in the house, whether private or pauper, together with notices of discharges, causes of death and also date of admissions. The emphasis was on compliance with the regulations rather than any malpractice towards the patients: 'These Statutes he is required to keep in his asylum, they are easily procured at the Queen's printers and will fully instruct him in the duties incumbent as the proprietor of a lunatic asylum.'[221]

In November 1841, the Secretary of State required the completion of an official return. Information required included details of the number of patients and the number of visits which had been made by officials of the court over the past five years, 1836-1840. Symes had made no such returns of either admissions, deaths or removals to the Clerk of the Peace; the return was blank. No medical visitor appeared to have attended although one had been appointed. Two visitations were made in 1839 and five in 1840. No licences had been regularly obtained, and in consequence considerable arrears were due from him. It was a series of administrative failures for which Symes had no ready answer. A notice of a motion was given to prosecute him for operating without a licence.[222]

William Symes somehow continued to manage the asylum, but with some restrictions as was minuted by the court in October 1842, when upon his licence renewal application Lord Shaftesbury moved that the licence be renewed on payment of £20, being £5 for the previous year and £15 for the current year. Mr Sturt seconded the motion and with 19 members in support and only three in opposition the motion was carried.[223]

At the time Symes wrote to Mr Fooks with copy of the reports of the visiting magistrates who had inspected the house the previous year. there was an air of desperation in the letter asking for a renewal of his licence for three male patients and three female patients:

it is my intention to be at Dorchester on Tuesday 18. I shall leave here early in the morning and get to Dorchester by 11 or 12 o'clock. I will go directly to

221   DCH, Q/A/L/Private/3.
222   Ibid.
223   DHC, Q/S/M/1/17, f. 241.

the hall and shall be ready for answer to my name being called any time after the times above named.

It appears that Cranborne was simply too small and had too few patients for commercial viability. This was compounded by a catalogue of administrative failures by Symes and the end of 1842 the Justices of the Peace were not particularly well disposed towards him. The asylum at Cranborne had run its course, but Symes would continue to be involved in the asylum business.

FORSTON

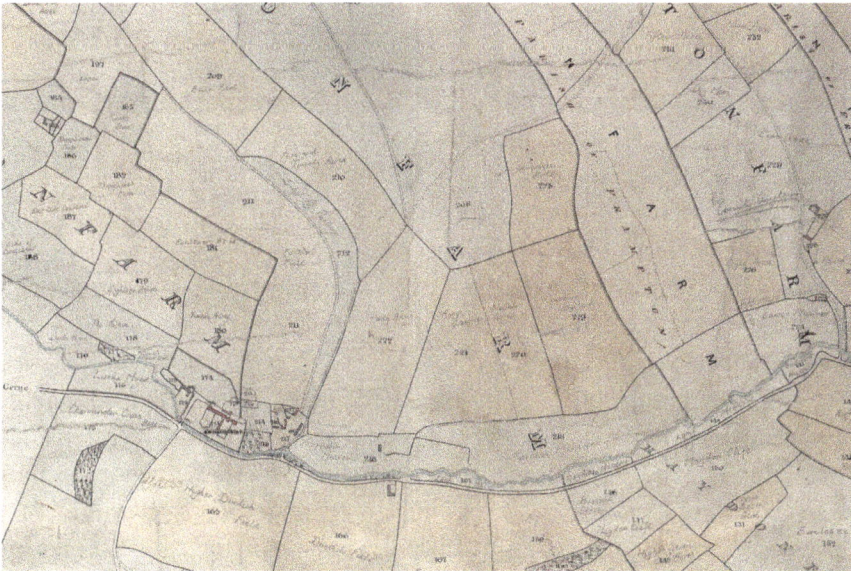

Section of Charminster tithe map, 1839, showing the asylum at Forston (bottom left, number 174) which was described in the accompanying apportionment as the Asylum Gardens and Premises covering an area in excess of eight acres. It is occupied by 'Lunatics' and owned by 'The Magistrates of the County of Dorset for the Time Being'. The site of the proposed asylum at Herrison (top/centre right, number 229).

MOVES WERE MADE in 1828 to build Dorset's public asylum.[224] In this aspect Dorset was ahead of the game as it was not until 1845 when the building of asylums became compulsory.[225] The process may have been

224   DHC, Q/S/M/1/16.

225   Parry-Jones, *The Trade in Lunacy*, p.16.

prompted by the generous gift of property and seven acres of land from local MP Francis John Browne. His intention was to 'relieve the County from the expense of purchasing land', and some of the building costs, by donating a house called Forston House. It included adjoining outhouses, garden and a field for 'use of the County for ever'. He also gave £4,000 in stocks towards its endowment.[226] If there were objections to the planned site they were not recorded; it would have been an offer difficult to turn down.

Alongside this objective the Quarter Sessions record, in January 1828, the appointment of 'Visiting Justices to Superintend the construction ... and also the management of such Lunatic Asylum'.[227] They were expected to report on its progress to the court and other affairs at various times.

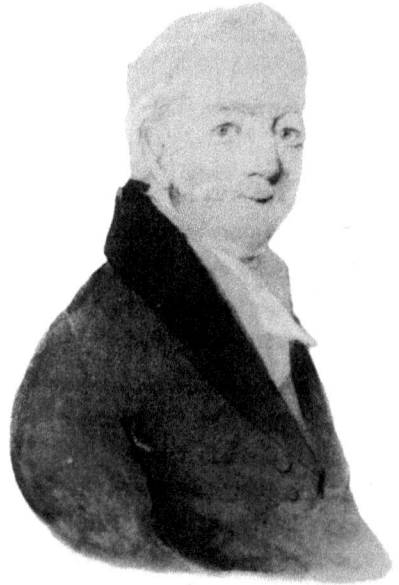

Francis John Browne MP who donated Forston house to the county for use as an asylum. Copyright West Dorset Mental Health NHS Trust, April 1992

Of the group some had prior experience of the workings of lunatic asylums which, in particular, was Halstock. The first Justice to visit Halstock was John Wyldbore Smith in 1809 and again in 1812; he would become High Sheriff of Dorset in 1814. Sir William Oglander, High Sheriff in 1817, also visited in 1816, 1819 to 1822 and 1824. Francis John Browne was another early visitor who went to Halstock each year more than any other Justice from 1810 to 1817. Perhaps observations made during these times provided the catalyst which empowered him to do something significant. In 1828 two additional Justices, Robert Gordon and John White, also known to Halstock, were appointed. All would have brought their expertise to the proposed asylum at Forston.

Notice was to be given in the usual newspapers that it was the intention of the Justices of the Peace to consider the provision of a Lunatic

226   DHC, Q/S/M/1/16. f.54
227   Ibid., f.53

Dorsetshire

A Return of the Number of Lunatics and Idiots within the said County taken from the Returns delivered by the Clerks to Justices of the Peace acting within the said County pursuant to an Order of Epiphany Session 1828.

Divisions	Number of Lunatics	Number of Idiots	Total Number	Dangerous
Dorchester	14	12	26	2
Bridport	18	26	44	7
Blandford ..	11	4	15	1
Wareham....	12	6	18	1
Sherborne ..	8	3	11	4
Wimborne ...	11	13	24	5
Cerne	2	11	13	2
Sturminster ..	8	10	18	2
Shaston ..	15	13	28	8
Total	**99**	**98**	**197**	**32**

Survey made in response to an order from the Quarter Sessions in January 1828 to ascertain who may be 'proper objects for a Lunatic Asylum'. This document shows the results of an attempt to provide the 'exact' numbers of lunatics living in the nine Dorset parish unions. DHC, Q/A/L

Asylum in the county in pursuance of the 1828 Act.[228] Those present were Charlton Byam Wollaston, chairman, Sir Robert Steele, knight and James Frampton. Thanks were to be presented to Francis John Browne for his 'well judged donation'. The Justices of the Peace were 'fully convinced of the infinite benefit which will accrue to all the unfortunate persons who may be the objects of this charity' and which will lessen the burden on the parishes by providing proper accommodation, care and medical treatment for those in need.

228   DHC, NG-HH/CMR/1/4/1.

Alongside the general construction and setting up of the new asylum an attempt was made to establish numbers of lunatics present in the county.[229] Therefore, in January 1828 at the Epiphany Sessions, an order was made to the clerks of the nine parish union divisions to supply, in time for the next Quarter Sessions, the number of of lunatics and idiots who 'may appear to be imperfect' and who may be 'proper objects for a Lunatic Asylum'. Those who were considered dangerous were also noted. The resulting return proved to be less than accurate but it was a measure of sorts which no doubt provided some idea as to the provision required at Forston.

The considerable financial donation of £4,000 was put into a trust, the dividends from which were to pay for a surgeon and matron at the asylum.[230] Further funds were raised by loans and the County Rate with £3,000 arising from voluntary subscription.[231]

Forston House, was situated just outside Charminster, a small village within easy reach of Dorchester, the county town. The house, soon to be the pauper lunatic asylum needed to be altered and furnishings supplied in order for it to be fit to receive patients and, in view of the returns made from a number of parishes, the number of patients was to be at least 40.[232] William Evans was appointed to survey the property and to confer with Dr Finch of Salisbury, the proprietor of Laverstock and Fisherton asylums, as to its best adaptation with the probability in mind that some rooms may be needed for 'patients of a superior class'. He was also instructed to visit Dr Finch's asylums, produce a plan with estimate and deliver it to the Visiting Justices of the Peace in Blandford, August 1828. Dr Finch, as 'superintendent of a very extensive establishment' who was thought to have 'much knowledge and experience on the subject' was asked to view the property and offer advice. The asylum's capacity was raised again to take 60 patients once the building plans had been approved.[233]

Prior to the opening of the asylum on 1 August 1832, the Visitors recommended the public be notified by an advertisement in the county newspapers. Overseers of the poor in each parish were to receive notice to provide an official return to the Clerk of the Peace, making known the number of those insane and chargeable to their parish. Failure to do so would incur a penalty of £10. It was the intention that each case of insanity

229   DHC, Q/S/M/1/16, f.53.

230   DHC, NG-HH/CMR/1/4/1.

231   Brown, *History of Dorset Hospitals*, p.169.

232   DHC, NG-HH/CMR/1/4/1.

233   Rogers, *In the Course of Time*, p.15

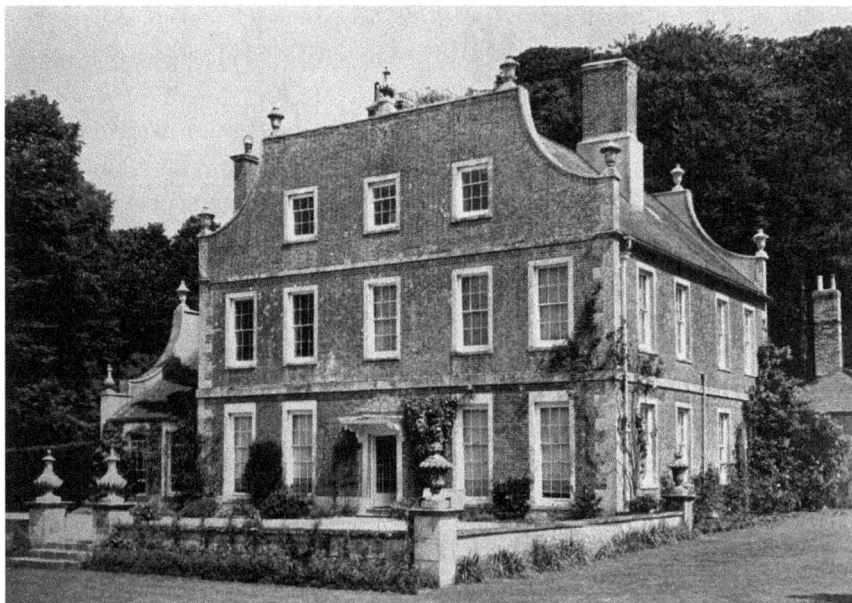

Forston house, site of the first Dorset county asylum. Crown copyright.

would be examined by the Justices in preparation for their admittance to Forston.[234]

By the October of 1832, two months after the asylum opened, it was clear that compliance in following these instructions was failing and stated that the Justices 'have experienced a considerable degree of backwardness' from parish officers.[235] This had resulted in a far less than expected number of patients admitted and in contrast to the information gathered from the annual returns. The cause for this reluctance was primarily the greater cost to the parish; the workhouse or staying at home prevailed until no longer viable.[236]

From the beginning the asylum at Forston was designed for pauper patients, but there were a number of various groups, or classes, within its original concept. On a visit made by C. B. Wollaston in October 1832 he noted that the

lower galleries, where the windows were darkened so as to admit of less air were intended for patients only of a more violent description. It seems

234 DHC, NG-HH/CMR/1/4/1.

235 Ibid.

236 Brown, *History of Dorset Hospitals*, p.173.

desirable that the upper galleries, where there is not the same objection of wants of light and air, should be used by the better kind of patients.[237]

He went on to say that there are not enough staff to divide them (the different classes) between the different galleries. Attention turned to providing a definition of an 'idiot'.[238] The Visitors reported that one distinction may be made between 'dangerous or mischievous and such as are harmless and occasionally employed in some work'. Such patients were not be be accommodated close to other paupers which caused additional distress. It was recognised that removing them from a previous situation of a 'crowded houses set apart for the poor' would be significant in securing a cure and subsequent release.

From August 1832 until the end of the year 23 people were admitted to Forston. All apart from one were from Dorset and according to their admission papers all were capable of self-harm or had caused injury to others. Two of these were from Halstock: Martha Dunford and James Wellstead.[239] Two women had been sent from Dorchester gaol, acquitted of their crimes due to insanity. The violent insane, whether from the workhouse or private asylum, took some precedence in securing a place at Forston. It appears that no patients were admitted from Stockland at this time.

Visits to Forston by appointed Justices of the Peace continued in much the same manner as the private asylums. Except perhaps, with a small yet important change, the ensuing reports were keen to reflect a positive approach particularly in respect of the asylum proprietor. This was demonstrated in 1838 where it was 'with much pleasure' to meet the superintendent Mr Quick and his wife, the matron, Mrs Quick. This sense of goodwill continued, the Visitor's said, even when faced with visits at unexpected times, they always found the patients and building in good order.[240]

In January 1835 the Visitors reported to the magistrates at the Quarter Sessions of the 'continued prosperity and good management of this excellent Institution'.[241] It had been operating for two years and five months. Although optimism and investment in the project was generally held firm by the Visitors there was palpable disappointment in reporting that were

237   DHC, NG-HH/CMR/1/1/1.
238   DHC, NG-HH/CMR/1/4/1.
239   DHC, NG-HH/CMR/4/32A/015.
240   DHC, NG-HH/CMR/2/1/2.
241   Ibid.

Since the Opening of the Asylum on the 1st August, 1832, the number of Patients that have been Admitted amounts to 222, of whom 79 have been Discharged Cured, 3 as Improper objects, 41 have Died, and 99 now remain, 89 of whom being Aged Persons, or those who have been afflicted for a length of time, must be deemed Incurable.

At the opening of the Asylum, the Rate charged for the Maintenance of the Patients, was 9s. 11d. per Week, but it has been gradually reduced to 6s. 5d. at which sum it at present remains, the price of Provisions not allowing of a further reduction.

This decrease of Expence has been caused *first* by a greater number of Patients in the House, as nearly the same establishment is required for a small number as for a large one, and *secondly* by the employment of the Patients in the domestic Establishment, in the Kitchen Garden, and in the several Trades, which now furnish articles made in the House, at the mere cost price of the materials, which must otherwise have been purchased at a shop, at an increased value.

The House was originally built to hold 80 Patients, but by fitting up the upper rooms in the original dwelling-house, additional accommodation has been afforded for 20 Patients more, and since the new cells have been built, 115 can be admitted.

Forston patient statistics, fees and employment of patients, 1832-1838, as published in the Visiting Justices report book. DHC, NG-HH/CMR/2/1/2.

vacancies for four males and four females. This state of affairs had occurred despite returns made to the Clerk of the Peace that there were many people still in the community needing assistance.

Numbers gradually increased, perhaps in part due to the decrease in weekly fees from 9s. 11d at the outset to a greatly reduced new rate, reported in 1838, of 6s 5d.[242] At Halstock, 20 years earlier, the fee which excluded

242   Ibid.

clothing and medicine, was almost double at 12s. As result apartments were added to the attic and over the offices, providing increased accommodation in 1838 for 82, 40 females and 42 males.[243] The extra expense incurred was explained and justified stating that 'for every parish within the county is, and will continue to be, permanently interested and benefitted thereby'. By 1838 the asylum was able to take 115 patients.

The records contain information about staff salaries and in particular the Superintendent Mr Quick, expressed his wish in 1837 for a salary raise owing to the increased number of patients and his extra responsibilities.[244] He explained that he had found it necessary to pay from his salary £10 for someone to keep the accounts and another £3 extra to manage the patients. Mr Quick had done his homework as he related the fact that he received less than Superintendents in other asylums. Subsequently his salary was increased by £30 to £170, the matron received £50. It was noted that an increase in the patient weekly rate was not required.

Many people were employed in a range of useful occupations at Forston; it was a world away from the private asylums. A minimum of one attendant was required for every 25 patients who were tranquil and easy to manage.[245] One attendant at least for every 12 patients who were incontinent or displayed difficult behaviour. One attendant was to sleep in or be able to overlook each dormitory; there were no specific night staff. A chaplain was also appointed to look after the patients' spiritual needs who in 1833 was paid a salary of £50.

Considerable thought had apparently been put into the layout of the wards, perhaps as a result of advice received and also as a result of official visits made over the years to the private asylums and workhouses. The outcome of this was described in 1838 where provision had been made for 'noisy and refractory patients' towards the end of the male and female galleries. Much was made of the heating systems which were to warm the new cells for the unmanageable patients which would permeate through to the day rooms thus eliminating the need and cost of fuelling a fire.[246]

By 1840 eight new cells had been built providing additional accommodation for four males and four females in response to the rising number of incurable patients which were now filling the asylum.[247] Many had

243   Ibid.

244   Ibid..

245   Brown, *History of Dorset Hospitals,* p.169.

246   DHC, NG-HH/CMR/2/1/2.

247   Ibid.

been rejected. There was also a concern, echoing those raised at Stockland private asylum, that regulations concerning patient classification and the mixing of patients with diverse needs from the upper gallery and lower wards were being breached. The problem of managing the classification or separation of just two divisions of patients, males and females, within an asylum without any consideration of their conditions was raised by Dr Button in his supplementary report of 1843. At Forston he was critical of the lack of single rooms in which to accommodate patients who were 'liable to sudden excitement' or noisy at night. Such patients were disrupting the sleep of others, in dormitories of five or six, often for several hours. He said for those requiring a quiet environment, such as in cases of sickness, the arrangement of the rooms was likely to inhibit recovery.

At the same time as the provision of additional accommodation an 'open shed' had been constructed nearer to the wards in which straw was to be kept for the 'dirty' patients. This had previously been stored at some distance from the main building which when moved inside during wet weather rendered it 'not in that dry state in which it ought to be'. It was also recognised that the shed offered further possibilities as an area in which additional patient employment could take place in wet conditions. It could be concluded that not providing a proper place to keep bedding straw dry demonstrated a lack of sensible planning, perhaps overlooked completely. Loose straw continued to be used as bedding until 1852.[248] The report also revealed the acute attention made to every cost and that every opportunity was taken to use patients as plentiful labour.

Only a few months after Forston opened its doors the heating systems, pipework, fittings and stoves were presenting areas for concern. In December 1832 the superintendent reported that the bath in the women's ward was leaking and unfit. The only option was to use the bath in the male quarters; it was reported still unusable in January 1833.[249]

It appeared that provision of personal care facilities generally were woefully inadequate and mismanaged. This, despite the recognition that bathing was beneficial by this time, the Visitors having suggested Halstock asylum provide a bath in 1828. A failing water closet in the female ward was also reported in January 1833 just 17 months after opening; concerns relating to the expense involved had prevented it being fixed. Eight years later the water closets were failing to work properly, perhaps due to the high numbers of patients coupled with poor building skills and general

248   Brown, *History of Dorset Hospitals,* p.171.
249   DHC, NG-HH/CMR/1/1/1.

inefficiency.[250] Visitor reports contain much of ongoing repairs and were usually proactive in dealing with problems raised by staff, such as agreeing with the fixing of shelves in an area where the clothing would not be exposed to damp.

A further concern was reported by Richard Sheridan one of the Visitors who had also been critical of conditions at Halstock. He expressed great surprise that the bed linen in the upper wards, for clean patients, was changed only once a month. He directed a change to fortnightly without delay whilst conceding the situation would be improved once the full quota of linen had arrived at the asylum.

By 1841 the property itself, despite its early promise, was beginning to present structural problems and in particular it was found to be damp. This was in part due to its low lying position and perhaps to a larger degree defective building work which had been hampered probably by continual cost cutting. Specifically the bricks had been laid as flooring directly on the earth in the lower wards which subsequently held water. This problem was exacerbated from the 'frequent washings' in respect of the 'worst class of patients'.[251] A new floor was required. Some improvements were made to the heating systems; pipes were installed to extend from the boiler in the kitchen to give some warmth to the patient wards.[252]

Ventilation issues were reported in January 1841 this being another area frequently mentioned by the Visitors to the private asylums. It appears some windows were not fitted with hinges which would allow them to be opened.[253] Windows and their frames were also failing, allowing the winter weather into the sleeping areas adding, no doubt, to the general damp atmosphere.

Two years later the Visitor's stated that the now crowded asylum was in urgent need of additional single cells and the provision of an infirmary. [254]Many diagnosed with recent 'attacks of lunacy' were being denied a place, knowledge of which had led to the proposal of adding further accommodation over the kitchen. At a later meeting this proposal was dismissed, recognising that adding an additional structure to the fragile old walls would not be expedient. Instead plans were made to add 20 beds to the current female wing and 16 additional rooms in the male wing of the building.

250   DHC, NG-HH/CMR/1/1/1.
251   DHC, NG-HH/CMR/1/4/1.
252   DHC, NG-HH/CMR/2/1/2.
253   DHC, NG-HH/CMR/1/1/1.
254   DHC, NG-HH/CMR/1/4/1.

The county asylum patients were employed in useful occupations unless they were said to be incapable. This was in contrast to the private asylums where very little provision was made for patients to work. In 1838 Mr Quick, the superintendent, was said to be proactive in his adopted approach to employing patients in many tasks, some relating to their previous trade. Unsurprisingly results were good said to be beneficial to the patients, whose recovery was being aided, and to the asylum itself.[255] The value of occupational therapy had been realised.[256]

Trades mentioned included tailors and shoemakers, patients were even entrusted with the tools required such as knives and hammers; no accidents had occurred at this time. Outside tradesmen were employed to teach and assist in these activities the results of which were sold or made use of within the asylum and at the gaol. Outside help was was hired for supervising work in the kitchen garden the produce of which was used in the asylum. It was reported that despite the garden being outside the walls of the asylum and employing up to 12 patients at a time, only one patient had escaped during the year. Other works undertaken by patients were labouring jobs such as digging foundations for new buildings and levelling ground.

The women were employed in the laundry and kitchen and general domestic duties. They knitted worsted stockings both for use in the asylum and to sell elsewhere. As a result, the Visitors reported that the need for hiring staff had been lessened by the work being done by the patients. This activity and employment of patients made way for a lower, perhaps unexpected, maintenance rate which inevitably benefitted all Dorset parish communities. At the turn of the decade, in December 1840, there were 47 out of 59 patients occupied in some sort of work. Six were unemployed and a further six patients were sick.[257]

Dr Button wrote in his report of 1841 that any small profit made from the work was used to buy tea and tobacco for the patients who '*thus commendably exert themselves*'.[258]This money was also set aside to assist patients at the time of their discharge. Dr Button suggested that in line with other county asylums the setting up of a charitable fund would be beneficial to '*enliven the too often gloomy prospect*' of a patient, perhaps destitute, returning home.

255   DHC, NG-HH/CMR/2/1/2.

256   Brown, *History of Dorset Hospitals,* p.171.

257   DHC, NG-HH/CMR/1/4/1.

258   DHC, NG-HH/CMR/2/1/2.

CHARITABLE FUND.

The following is a list of the Donations and Subscriptions received from the establishment of the Charitable Fund, for the relief of persons discharged from the Asylum, who are considered suitable objects. The money has been placed in the Dorchester Saving's Bank, from which it is drawn as wanted.

		£	s.	d.
1842—Sir R. Glyn	(annual)	5	0	0
Rev. Carr Glyn	(annual)	1	0	0
Rev. W. Cutler		1	0	0
W. Devenish, Esq.	(annual)	1	0	0
J. Henning, Esq.		0	10	0
1843—R. Williams, Esq.		2	0	0
Hon. Mrs. G. Damer		1	0	0
Rev. W. Churchill		1	0	0
Hon. and Rev. S. G. Osborne	(annual)	1	1	0
Rev. Carr Glyn		1	0	0
R. B. Sheridan, Esq., M.P.		2	0	0
Sir R. Glyn		5	0	0
A. H. D. Acland, Esq.		1	0	0
J. Floyer, Esq., M.P.		1	0	0
Collected after Sermon at Frampton Church		12	6	10
Rev. J. A. Templer		0	10	0
Rev. C. Bingham		0	10	0
Mrs. Mary Frampton		1	0	0
The Right Hon. the Earl of Shaftesbury	(annual)	5	0	0
W. P. Hodges, Esq.		0	10	0
Mrs. G. Bankes		1	0	0
Rev. W. Cutler		1	0	0
Geo. Harris, Esq.		1	0	0
Sale of Sermons by Rev. C. Bingham		2	3	0
1844—Miss Jackson	(annual)	1	0	0
Rev. C. Bingham		0	10	0
Rev. Carr Glyn		1	0	0
The Right Hon. the Earl of Shaftesbury		5	0	0
Mrs. Mary Frampton		1	0	0
Charles Porcher, Esq.		5	0	0
Rev. J. A. Templer		1	0	0
Col. Damer, M.P.		1	0	0
1845—Rev. C. Bingham		0	10	0
Miss Jackson		1	0	0
Hon. and Rev. — Scott		0	10	0
A Friend		5	0	0
Rev. Carr Glyn		1	1	0
Rev. W. Cutler		1	0	0
R. M. Milnes, Esq., M.P.		0	10	0
Hon. and Rev. S. G. Osborne		1	0	0
Barrington Brown, Esq.		2	0	0
J. Cree, Esq.		0	10	0
1846—Subscriptions at Frampton House		8	0	0
Barrington Brown, Esq.		1	0	0
1847—Rev. Carr Glyn		1	0	0
1848—Mrs W. Williams		0	10	0
Lady Ellis		0	10	0
1849—Rev. J. A. Templer		0	10	0
Mrs. W. Williams		0	10	0
Rev. Carr Glyn		1	0	0
Sir R. Glyn		6	0	0
		£ 97	1	10

By relief afforded to 104 Patients during the same period　　　　　　　　　　　　£ 58　5　0

By Balance at the Bank　　　　　　　£ 38 16 10

Contributors to the charitable fund as published in the Visiting Justices report book covering the years 1842-1849. Brian Proctor and Samuel Gaskill, Lunacy Commissioners, expressed their pleasure on discovering that most of the Dorset Justices subscribed every year to this fund. It was designed to help patients upon leaving the asylum who had 'conducted themselves well and industriously' and also to those who required necessities of some urgency. DHC, NG-HH/CMR/2/1/2.

Visitors to the private asylums mentioned on occasion that they found patients occupying themselves by reading. At Forston, more interest was shown in this activity. In 1841 they reported that a few books had been provided at a cost of £5, but as yet they had been little used. On the other hand the prayer books and bibles were read on Sundays with some attentiveness. One report noted that a patient had been taught to read by others.[259]

As at the private asylums regulations required divine service to be offered and actively pursued every Sunday. At Forston even when the asylum opened in 1832 the room designated as a chapel was too small, accommodating just 40 patients including four servants.[260] Given the level of attention shown towards delivering this activity to patients elsewhere it is interesting to note that by 1841 the chapel was still not able to contain everyone who wished to attend. This was lamented by Dr Button where he also described in detail the 'degree of self control' displayed by patients who clearly gained much consolation from their attendance.

Records of patients at Forston were detailed and precise, perhaps reflecting the need for public accountability of the new institution. This represented a marked contrast to the level of record keeping at the three private asylums. Total numbers of patients remaining in the asylum at the end of each year are provided in Appendix 1 and the terms used to describe the diagnosis different classifications of patient in Appendix 4.

The importance of transparency and accountability was reflected in the detailed and regular reports made to the local press by the Quarter Sessions.[261] In January 1849 the Visiting Justices reported Forston's patient numbers and noted that over 50% had recovered and had been discharged on the admission of the year. Twelve patients had died, of which a significant proportion were of patients having been admitted in a 'weak state'; five had died within just three months of their admission. The reports demonstrated that while extolling the virtues of the general running of the asylum they did not shy away from reporting the difficulties encountered. These related primarily to the buildings which were in need of repair and estimates of the required funds were presented to readers. The newspaper also reported that the weekly rate for patients was to be raised from 7s. to 7s. 7d. 'in order to defray the charges of patients at Dr Finch's' whose establishment at Fisherton in Wiltshire was receiving chronic cases in order to free up space at Forston.

259 Ibid.. p.15
260 Ibid.
261 *Sherborne Mercury*, 6 January 1849.

13

A comparative table of cures, collected from reports of the various Asylums of the Kingdom, taken from the last Wakefield Report.

~~~~~~~~~~~~~~~~~~~~~~~~~~~~~~~

From 1796 to 1836, York Retreat, for the Society
of Friends,............ 46.45
1823 to 1833, Gloucester, 3 classes of patients
admitted, ... 45.34
1818 to 1838, Staffordshire, 3 do.   do... 44.9
1812 to 1838, Nottingham, 3 or 4 do.   do. 43.43
1820 to 1837, Lincoln, 3 do.   do...... 39.83
The Opening to 1839, Lancaster, 3 do. 38.83
1782 to 1839, Montrose, ... 39.26
1827 to 1838, Perth, opulent patients admitted 34.68
1814, to 1835, York, 4 classes of patients do. 31.5
To 1838, Glasgow, 3 do.   do............ 27.53
From 1836, to 1839, Dundee, 3 do.   do. 20.44

~~~~~~~~~~~~~~~~~~~~~~~~~~~~~

1818 to 1839, Wakefield, only paupers do... 43.92
Opening to 1839, Dorset, do.   do....... 41.0
1829 to 1838, Suffolk, do.   do......... 38.26
1836 to 1839, Edinburgh, do.   do..... 25.0
1831 to 1837, Hanwell, do.   do....... 20.98
1833 to 1837, Maidstone, do.   do....... 23.69

T. A. QUICK, M. D.

MEDICAL SUPERINTENDENT.

Table showing the per cent of patients cured at several asylums, 1782-1839. The management at Forston recognised that in order to uphold and increase support across the county much depended on the success of the institution which was largely measured by its cure rates. DHC, NG-HH/CMR/2/1/2.

Five levels of information were required which, in 1837, recorded admittance data from 1832 to 1837: there had been 45 cases not exceeding six months' duration, and first attack; 13 cases not exceeding twelve months' duration, and first attack; 10 cases not exceeding two years' duration and first attack; 107 cases of more than two years' duration and 47 cases of those who have had previous attacks, a total of 222 patients. This level of detail revealed the understanding, which was often minuted, that too many people were being admitted too late. However, the number admitted for six months or less seemed to be growing by this point, evidence perhaps that parish officials were recognising that early intervention was more likely to bring forward an early cure; resulting in less expense for the parish.

Similar detail was afforded to the discharges made from 1832 to 1837: 39 cases cured not having been insane more than six months before admission; six cases cured not having been insane more than twelve months before admission; 12 cases cured having been insane two years and upwards before admission; 22 cases cured having had previous attacks; there were five cases not cured, but discharged as improper objects (possibly a term used for those patients thought unlikely to be cured or 'idiots'). The total discharge number was 82.

During this period a record was maintained of the age range of the patients who had been discharged or died. From this information the group with the most admissions can be assigned to those between 40 and 50 years of age, a total of 57 patients. Under half of these, 22, were discharged and 13 died. The next largest group were people between 30 and 40 years of age. This group represented a slightly higher number of patients being discharged at 28 with only five deaths.

Continuing the theme that patients were presented for admission too late and therefore with virtually no hope of a cure the Visitors reported in 1840 that in the previous year 28 patients had arrived at Forston of whom only six considered to be curable.[262] The remainder, some from other asylums, were patients with longstanding illnesses and now thought to be incurable. The Visitors were concerned that the wording of the Act which mentioned 'dangerous lunatics, insane persons, and idiots' may be interpreted to mean that until a patient was perceived to be a danger to the life of another person they may be kept at home. They considered that keeping people in this way allowed the disease to become permanent with little optimism of a cure resulting in a burden on the parish for life. The outcome of this observation was to impress upon the magistrates to

262   DHC, NG-HH/CMR/2/1/2.

influence parish officials and explain the importance to intervene as soon as people showed symptoms of insanity. The Poor Law Amendment Act 1834 which prohibited any dangerous lunatic, insane person or idiot to remain in the workhouse for longer than 14 days, may not have made the expected impact.

The annual report made by the superintending physician Dr Button in 1843 for the Quarter Sessions, highlighted that officials, including medical men, often failed to understand who should be admitted to a lunatic asylum.[263] It appears that its primary purpose was considered to be for the 'furious maniac' or the 'lost and helpless idiot' who in reality only formed a small number of the really insane. There seems to have been little knowledge that insanity existed in many various degrees just as was the case in other diseases.

At the Easter Sessions, 1840, the Visitor's expressed concern that the asylum 'continues quite full'.[264] Construction of additional accommodation was to begin soon but in the short term attention was focussed on the possibility of removing three 'idiots' from the house to create further room. However, until a proper place had been secured for them in the Union Workhouse, or elsewhere, the Visitors were reluctant to discharge them. Their dilemma was that the idiots, whose cure was 'hopeless' were taking up places for those who may benefit and receive some relief from their illness.

In the summer sessions of 1840 the asylum was now declared completely full.[265] It appeared that the parish officials had overcome their reluctance to send people to Forston so much so that the Visitors found it necessary to strongly advise first checking availability. To stress the point reference was made of two patients from the west of the county, Lyme Regis and Bridport, and one from Axminster in Devon, who were turned away immediately after making the considerable journey to Charminster.

In discussing various cases the superintending physician Dr Button, explained in his year end report of 1841 that people who had been discharged and subsequently readmitted, sometimes several times, had remained at home between each episode.[266] His classification of the causes of the conditions of the patients at Forston with relative numbers of male and female patients is provided in Appendix 4. He believed that hereditary predisposition existed sometimes traceable back to the third generation and

263   DHC, NG-HH/CMR/2/1/2.

264   DHC, NG-HH/CMR/1/4/1.

265   Ibid.

266   DHC, NG-HH/CMR/2/1/2..

shared his opinion that the hereditary disposition to insanity was 'more distressful than in any other disease'. He continued

> (this) should be a warning against contracting inconsiderate marriages; this predisposition being increased by consanguinity (a close relationship) of the parents, and greatly aggravated by the union of two similarly vitiated (impaired) constitutions.

Other causes of mental illness particularly noted were grief, anxiety, domestic misery and injury to the head. [267] But, he was keen to stress that in total contrast to other county asylums not one person had been admitted in the past year with intemperance given as the cause. He expressed the hope that his demonstrated some improvement 'in the moral state of the county'. He said the majority of patients suffered from chronic dementia, little could be done except help with regular habits and cleanliness and provide amusement and some occupation where possible.[268]

Patients were usually 'removed' to the county asylum due to cost: funds either having been exhausted or simply because it was a cheaper option. Other contributing factors included the provision of the necessary care for managing extreme behaviour which was more difficult in the smaller private institutions and for which few people had the appropriate skills. The impact of this change must have been significant, possibly welcomed by asylum proprietors on occasion, perhaps freeing up places for less challenging patients. There is no suggestion that the wishes of the patients, or their families, were taken into consideration when they were transferred between institutions.

The Quarter Session documents did not always show a direct move from Halstock or Stockland to Forston. Sometimes there was a gap of some years between leaving a private asylum and admittance to the county asylum. Patients were often 'removed' by family and taken home only to be found at Forston in later years. Isaac Cooper was said to be 'cured' when he was removed from Halstock by his brother in 1829, but he was admitted to Forston in 1841 when he was said to be insane through contracting typhus.[269]

Between the years 1832 and 1848 at least 25 pauper patients had been admitted from Halstock to Forston out of a total of 64 identifiable pauper

267 Ibid. p.10.
268 Ibid. p.13.
269 DHC, NG-HH/CMR/4/32A/053.

patient admissions during the same period. The highest number were transferred in the first three years, including seven in 1832. By 1843, when it had been open for 11 years, Forston held 113 patients from across the country.

Providing affordable and secure care for the insane poor was the primary consideration of parish officials, it was their responsibility to contain and reduce, where possible, payments made from the parish poor rates. Parish records of Buckland Newton show the charge for Martha Porter was 7s. 7d. in 1835.[270] This figure, fixed by the asylum's official Visitors, included maintenance and care, medicine and clothing and the salaries of staff. However, it appears the parishes were expected to pick up the bill for funeral and coffin expenses as was the case at Buckland Newton where legal proceedings were threatened unless £4 12s. was paid for two of their pauper parishioners who had died at Forston.

The record keeping at Forston in relation to patient diagnosis and treatment was far more detailed than at the private asylums. The order papers, drawn up at the admission of each new patient, also provide biographical details of the patients from which it is possible to examine the situations some of those patients who had previous been incarcerated elsewhere. Forston asylum, received only about nine patients from Stockland asylum at the time of its closure. Another four had previously been released from Stockland where they were 'cured', but were admitted to Forston shortly afterwards.

The low number Stockland patients admitted to Forston was most likely due to over subscription. It had been built to accommodate just 60 patients and was soon overwhelmed. A report by the Visiting Justices to Forston in 1839 was published in the local newspaper, they stated that

> the number of patients without hope cure had increased' and that the asylum was kept constantly full, that admittance had, during the past quarter, been necessarily refused to several applications.

It was suggested that only enlarging the building would solve the difficulty. A total of 106 patients were resident in Forston in 1839.[271] Part of the problem was that Devon county asylum would not open until 1845, so several patients were initially transferred back to Devon parishes and union workhouses before their mental health conditions meant that they were

270   DHC, PE-BCN/OV/3/5.
271   *Dorset County Chronicle* 17 October 1839.

eventually moved to Forston. One former Stockland patient, William Wills, was admitted to Forston in January 1842, with two letters of transfer from Seaton in Devon.[272] Another, William Cross, was transferred with similar papers from Axminster union in the same month.[273]

Although the record keeping at Forston was meticulous a patient's earlier incarceration in Stockland was not always recorded; perhaps because it had not been revealed. The entry for Mary Farrant, admitted January 1842, in the case register noted that she was from Axminster, aged 55, married and was literate. Her first attack was at the age of 30 and she had suffered repeated attacks since that time; dementia was noted, but no details of her earlier spell at Stockland was provided. She was buried at Charminster aged 71.[274]

Another former Stockland patient, Peter Tolman, had married in Chideock, where he was resident, in 1822.[275] In 1829 he was admitted and confined for less than six months before his discharge, 'on trial', in December. By 1831 he had been readmitted and remained until another discharge in 1833. In the census of 1841, an agricultural labourer now living in Allington with Harriet his wife and eight children. But by 1845 Peter was admitted to Forston stating that he had been insane for 12-14 years, was epileptic and a danger to others.[276] Two years later he was buried in Charminster aged 57.[277]

Occasionally patients had left Stockland for admittance to Forston in previous years when the two institutions were running in parallel with each other, although the records rarely confirm a direct move. At Forston they were just as likely to be discharged as cured and later readmitted as they had been at Stockland. Mary Cookney of Lyme Regis was such a case, having first been confined at Stockland in 1832. By February 1833 she had been discharged, said to be cured. She was admitted to Forston in 1834 described as pauper, 40 years old, a servant and single. Her cause of insanity was unknown, but she displayed violent tendencies and had threatened to injure people. There had been a 'previous attack in poorhouse'. She was said to be 'religious and given to talk much'. The Forston staff noted that she had been confined twice at Stockland and

272   DHC, NG-HH/CMR/4/32B/337 and NG-HH/CMR/4/32B/339.
273   DHC, NG-HH/CMR/4/32B/338.
274   DHC, PE-CMR/RE/4/1.
275   DHC, PE-CDK/RE/3/2.
276   DHC, NG-HH/CMR/4/32B/491.
277   DHC, PE-CMR/RE/4/1.

discharged on both occasions having been considered cured.[278] Mary was discharged from Forston in April 1835, again believed to have been cured.[279] But, by January 1841 Mary had been re-admitted to Forston. She was said to be threatening to others although of good temper, she was 'fond of nursing', and her condition was thought to be hereditary. [280]She was again released in June 1841, having been cured, but readmitted by the Axminster Union in February of 1843 [281] Mary died in November 1859 and was buried, like so many other patients, at Charminster.

Pauper patients were also removed from Halstock to the newly opened county asylum at Forston. In August 1832 James Wellstead was removed from Halstock to Forston. At the same time the Visitors at Halstock also stated that Robert Childs 'should be taken away as there appears to be no reason why he should be confined in a Lunatic asylum'. Yet shortly afterwards, in January 1833, an order paper shows a Robert Childs of Whitcombe admitted to Forston, aged 53 years old.[282] He had been in Halstock for less than a year. Martha Dunford, aged 40, from Abbotsbury was also moved to Forston in its first year of opening. Her cure prognosis at Halstock had been described as 'doubtful' so perhaps she was removed for a second opinion. Her Forston order papers state that she had four children, no occupation, was sometimes violent, disposed to self harm and had the potential to injure others.[283] Her death was recorded in 1849 aged 57 at Forston.[284] She was returned to Abbotsbury for burial where the parish records made no mention of either asylum.[285]

Hannah Young from Cattistock suffered from various mental health problems. She was a domestic servant who was admitted to Halstock by the Cattistock overseers in July 1831. Some alternative provision had been found for her care when she was relieved and discharged, in the October of that year, only to be readmitted by December. Four years later she was sent to Forston, aged 72. Her order paper described her as having been insane for 15 years partly due to her master's suicide and partly out of fear of 'being

278   DHC, NG-HH/CMR/4/32A/112.

279   DHC, NG-HH/CMR/4/1/3.

280   DHC, NG-HH/CMR/4/32B/304.

281   DHC, NG-HH/CMR/4/32B/377.

282   DHC, NG-HH/CMR/4/32A/047.

283   DHC, NG-HH/CMR/4/32A/016.

284   DHC, NG-HH/CMR/4/10A/1.

285   DHC, PE-ABB/RE/4/1.

reduced to want in intelligence'. Her temperament alternated between passive and violent and she had attempted suicide twice.[286] Charminster parish register recorded her burial in May 1837, aged 74, complete with a note that she was from the 'lunatic asylum'.[287] Many patients were buried at Charminster rather than their home parish and, as with Hannah Young, identified as inmates of Forston.

The demand for places was high and easily outstripped supply which meant that Forston used the private asylums for overflow patients. In December 1839 when two people were admitted to Halstock because Forston was full. One of these was Job Warren who was said to be 22 years old, although his baptism records indicate that he was older.[288] His father was a blacksmith and he was a labourer from Tincleton. He remained at Halstock for a year until a place became available at Forston a year later in December 1840. His admission paper stated that there was no known specific cause for his state of mind, but that he suffered from epilepsy.[289] His name was included in the 1841 census records for Forston, where his occupation was given as a 'thresher'.[290] The Forston records show that he was released having been cured in June 1841.[291] His burial was registered in 1844 at Tincleton when he was aged 28.[292]

Before the county asylum was constructed at Forston criminal lunatics were placed in private asylums, Joseph Whiterow of Kimmeridge who was confined at Halstock is given as one of the case studies. Many were transferred out of Dorset, particularly to Fisherton, in Wiltshire. The following people were identified as criminal lunatics and confined at Forston. None had had previously been incarcerated at Halstock or Stockland.

A letter from Whitehall in December 1836 to Mr Fooks, Clerk of the Peace, concerned Thomas Randall and Edith Still who were both incarcerated at Forston asylum:

> although these persons are certified to be sane his Lordship cannot but entertain some doubt whether it would be safe at the present time to dismiss

286 DHC, NG-HH/CMR/4/32A/116.

287 DHC, PE-CMR/RE/4/1.

288 DHC, PE-TIN/RE/1/2.

289 DHC, NG-HH/CMR/4/32A/303.

290 *Census* 1841.

291 DHC, NG-HH/CMR/4/1/3.

292 DHC, PE-TIN/RE/3/1.

them and leave them to their own disposal. If inconvenient to keep them propose to remove them back to the gaol from where they came.[293]

The more serious of the two, Thomas Randall aged 45, was charged at Winchester with the wilful murder of his wife Elizabeth Randall, in Portsea, warrant dated 1831. He was acquitted on the grounds of insanity and to be kept in strict custody until His Majesty's pleasure be known.[294] Revd G Pickard petitioned the Winchester Lent Assizes in 1832 for his removal to Forston which would lessen the expense to Wareham parish.[295] Further documents confirm his acquittal at the Hampshire Lent Assizes in 1832.[296]

Edith Still was admitted to Forston in August 1832 from Dorchester gaol.[297] Originally from the parish of Fontmell Magna she was acquitted of a criminal offence, arson, on the grounds of insanity.[298]

However, in December 1836, a warrant was prepared for the removal from Forston asylum of both Randall and Still back to the county gaol as they were no longer considered insane.[299]

In April 1837 Edith Still's case was considered in a lengthy letter written by C B Wollaston (Visiting Justice to the Gaol)[300] to the Home Office where it was requested that if she could not be pardoned she should be removed from Dorchester gaol and returned to Forston.[301] Wollaston stated that Edith had been reported as sane for three years by Forston's medical superintendent and that an application had been made, in November 1836, for her discharge. A month later a response was received from the Secretary of State which expressed doubt that it would be safe to discharge her but if it was inconvenient to keep her at the asylum she should be returned to the gaol. Before any reply was made to the London office, Edith was taken back to prison. Wollaston, (in his additional role as a Visiting Justice to Forston)[302], declared his belief that if a person was pronounced 'perfectly

293   DHC, Q/A/L/Criminal/1/1.

294   TNA. PCOM 2/418 and 2/421.

295   TNA, HO 17/114/39, 1832.

296   TNA, HO 27/44, f.298.

297   DHC, NG-HH/CMR/4/32A/007.

298   TNA, HO 13/60, f.324.

299   TNA, HO 17/114/39, 1832.

300   DHC, Q/S/M/1/17, 1836-1845.

301   TNA, HO 17/36, 1837.

302   DHC, Q/S/M/1/16, 1827-1836.

sane' they should be placed under the care of 'friends' and not occupy a place required for an insane patient at the asylum (nor presumably in gaol). He also emphasised that there had been no 'difficulty as to the room for her' in 1836 or at the present time at Forston. Furthermore, he conveyed that her health had suffered since the strict regime of confinement in the prison. The prison's surgeon also contributed that her mind had not been helped by the lack of air and exercise as well as a difference in the food. It seems Edith was able to talk 'rationally' about her cause of detention and 'present feelings'.

The content of this letter demonstrates the very real dilemmas presented to the court by people who committed crimes, often serious, who were believed insane and the extent of moving people from one place of incarceration to another. It also reveals the attention and consideration brought by those in power in order to seek the best outcome for many.

Edith's subsequent story remains unclear but it is possible that she was a boarder, aged 76, from Fontmill; in the house of Charles Richards as defined by the Canford census of 1861.

In answer to a request made from Whitehall in 1838 of those acquitted by the Quarter Sessions on account of insanity in last ten years, just two were named: Amelia Jeffries and Ambrose Cook. In 1843 Dr Button, Superintendent at Forston, responded to a request for the number of criminal lunatics confined at the asylum. His list again comprised just two: William Elliott, who had threatened the life of a person in 1841 and Matthew Clapp who had committed theft in 1839.[303]

Forston asylum was evidently over crowded and would struggle to accommodate the patients from the Devon parishes within the Axminster poor law union released on the closure of Stockland asylum. Although the Axminster union had failed to grasp the lack of capacity available in Dorset when Stockland closed the authority in Devon had already recognised the need for an institution within their own county. The situation was under discussion before Stockland's closure in a report presented to the Justices of the Peace at the Devon County Sessions in October 1839:

> My attention at this time is particularly drawn to it by a pamphlet which find placed here ("Thoughts on the present Distribution of the Pauper Lunatics") And will merely state my firm conviction, from knowledge which have derived in my situation as guardian under the Poor Laws, and in other ways, that it is essential to the interests of humanity, and even of economy, that some system — for now we have none — for the care and treatment

303   DHC, Q/A/L/Criminal/1/1.

of pauper lunatics should be adopted. You will remember the last year I suggested a mode that, as I thought, would have very much done away the objections which have been made to the establishment of a pauper lunatic asylum in this county, and that was by a slight alteration in the Poor Law Act have formed a Union of Unions for this purpose, the guardians being selected from the several Boards of Guardians. I believe it was only from accidental causes such alteration was not made in the act passed in the last Sessions, and I have reason to believe that at a very early period in the next Session that alteration will be made. These persons are now sent a distance and at a very great expense, to private asylums. l am very far from intending to say there is anything improper in private asylums, but this I do say, that seeing the proprietors look to them as a means livelihood and of profit to themselves, there is no private asylum that can afford that proper mode of treatment which is necessary for the restoration of the unhappy persons who are afflicted this way; and I do hope we shall lose no time in getting rid of this stigma on the county.[304]

Plans had been drawn up for an asylum in Exeter in 1829 in response to the 1828 Lunacy Act.[305] The Devon county asylum opened at Exminster with an initial capacity of 440 beds in 1845. No doubt the Devon authorities anticipated the success of the Dorset asylum at Forston and had taken note of the Dorset asylum's limited capacity.

In September 1842 the *Dorset County Chronicle* was complimentary in its assessment:

Lunatic asylum - At a meeting of the committee of the County Lunatic asylum held on Monday the 1st inst. two patients were discharged cured. This valuable institution, we are pleased to find is going on very prosperously, and promises to be productive of every good result anticipated from it. With reference to this establishment it may not be generally known that besides the advantage of a lower rate of charge than that made at private asylums, there are no extra charges for medicines and clothing, both of which are charged on the patients at the Private Establishments, but are here provided for out of the funds of the asylum.

In his report of 1850 Dr Button turned his attention to the troubling misapprehension entertained by some as to the costs of the insane poor under

304 *Sherborne Mercury* 21 October 1839.
305 A history of Devon County Mental Hospital, https://dcmh.exeter.ac.uk/

the care of the public asylum.[306] Views held from want of correct information were mistaken and a comparison between the asylum's weekly rate, charged to the parishes, would show that the maintenance, medicine, care, clothing and salaries of officers and servants versus the costs of maintaining the same in parish Unions would be almost as the asylum. Higher costs for heating and beneficial food provision were generally absorbed; the larger the daily average of patients the less expense incurred.

People were often brought into the county asylum in a frail state, some were elderly, some had been ill treated, some were malnourished and some were simply exhausted. Many died soon after their arrival. Blame for this situation was rarely apportioned, but in December 1842 the Visitor's, referred to four cases having been admitted suffering from ill treatment.[307] Dr Button, the Forston superintendent, was requested to write to the Beaminster Union in respect specifically of one of these, a woman, who according to the nurse accompanying her had been confined at the workhouse in a straight waistcoat for one month. This was exactly the sort of situation that the county asylum had been created to prevent. As long as parishes and poor law unions remained able to make decisions, based solely on cost, to place patients in workhouses and as lodgers these abuses would remain. The legislation introduced in the Lunacy Acts of 1843 and 1845 sought to ensure that every county had an adequate asylum for the reception of pauper patients.

306   DHC, NG-HH/CMR/2/1/2.
307   DHC, NG-HH/CMR/1/4/1.

The county asylum and the end of
Dorset Private Asylums from 1842

THE LUNACY ACT 1842 dictated that in addition to visits by local
Justice of the Peace, the newly appointed Metropolitan Commissioners
in Lunacy, a physician and barrister, were to inspect each asylum twice a
year. They were, amongst other changes, required to report on the use of
mechanical restraint and activities available to the patients.[308] This increased
scrutiny arrived at a time when the Dorset private asylums were already in a
state of transition. Stockland was no longer licenced and as only one patient
remained it did not fall within the orbit of the Commissioners. Cranborne
was in financial difficulties and its failure to maintain proper records meant
that licence renewal was by no means certain. Halstock had considerably
fewer patients than it had accommodated a decade earlier. But, the young
surgeon John Justinian Mercer, assisted by his wife and aunt, was in charge
of what appeared to be a well managed institution. The county asylum
at Forston had been established for a decade and was clearly successful.
However, was greatly over subscribed, had found it necessary to house
patients in other institutions, and had experienced numerous problems
with unsuitable or poorly constructed buildings.

Increased public awareness of the role of private asylums was
highlighted in 1844 when Robert Gordon, one of the Metropolitan
Commissioners and a Visitor at Halstock proposed that the public be
notified through newspapers of the 'Renewal or Grant' of private asylum's
licences. The motion was resolved and recorded by the Clerk of the Peace in
Dorset.

The Lunacy Act of 1845 saw the Metropolitan Commissioners
renamed Lunacy Commissioners and of these many were familiar. The
Commissioners were highly qualified physicians, surgeons and solicitors
often with knowledge and experience of the insane; they travelled in pairs,
one medical and one legal.

308   Brown, *History of Dorset Hospitals*, p.164.

Dorset was at the centre of reforms to the asylum system. Robert Gordon and the Earl of Shaftesbury had been instrumental in commissioning the lunacy reports that had formed the basis for the Acts passed in 1842 and 1845 and had strong links with the county. Perhaps for this reason Samuel Gaskell, Medical Supervisor at Lancaster asylum and known for both his work into the restraint of patients and his painstaking attention to detail visited Halstock on four occasions, as part of the programme of official visits, during the 1850s. He was much admired by Shaftesbury who appointed him as Medical Commissioner in Lunacy in 1849, the first with expertise in the role of Commissioner.[309]

HALSTOCK

THE METROPOLITAN COMMISSIONERS, who inspected the Halstock asylum at various times after October 1842, were made up of four legal men Robert Lutwidge, Brian Procter, James Mylne, John Hancock Hall and six physicians who were Samuel Gaskell, Robert Nairne, John Hume, Thomas Turner, James Prichard and James Wilkes. Of these Thomas Turner made the most visits; attending five times between 1847 and 1855. During the final 12 years that Halstock was a certified asylum it received visits from the Lunacy Commissioners on 21 occasions ending in 1858. The Justices of the Peace continued to attend the asylum at different times to the Metropolitan Commissioners. They included W. J. Goodden, Lord Stavordale (Stephen Fox-Strangways), Samuel Cox, John Goodden, George Harbin and John Blennerhassett.

In October 1842 John Justinian Mercer was the proprietor of the asylum which was now referred to as Portland House. There were some positive comments made by the Metropolitan Commissioners in Lunacy. On their inaugural visit Proctor and Hawkins, said that the

> patients in this house appear to be comfortable and not otherwise than cheerful, and with one or two exceptions, sufficiently cleanly in their persons. The house is very old and capable of much improvement. The furniture in the bed rooms appear to us to be rather scanty.

309 Royal College of Surgeons of England, *Plarr's Lives of the Fellows*, Royal College of Surgeons of England; Sources *British Medical Journal* 1886, I, 720, https://livesonline.rcseng.ac.uk accessed 26 August 2025)

They continued to report that with one exception 'the patients were allowed to mingle freely with the family'. This last observation indicated a changed approach.

In less than a year, during a visit in July, 1843, the view of two different Metropolitan Commissioners was more critical. They reported that one room was found to be in a 'very filthy condition and the adjoining yard as bad'. They continued to state that the house was ill adapted for its purpose, the upper floor sleeping rooms close to roof so must be cold and they objected to violent patients of opposite sex living so close to each other. Despite the concerns about the buildings the report they were content with the treatment of the patients. The report also stated that there were seven males and four females residing in the house 'all in good bodily health and to be kindly treated' with no restraints except two violent patients confined in separate rooms. The Commissioners made an observation relating to the status of patients, which had previously been unreported: 'the better class of male patients amuse themselves in reading and working in the garden'.

The Commissioner's inspection the following year (August 1844) reported some improvements had been made but considered the apartments were a long way from being comfortable or cheerful. They also said that in winter the rooms would be cold and gloomy. They commented on the fact that the 'passages [were] free from offensive smells' which was a regular observation during this time. Again a note was made regarding the activities available to the patients who were able to walk about in the garden and neighbourhood. Whether both private and pauper patients were afforded the same activities is not known, there are no specific references made in respect of the two different groups during these later years. Most of the pauper patients had been removed to Forston or elsewhere by 1844.

A further recommendation to Mr Mercer was to provide and display a plan of the premises as this had been a stipulation of the Act of 1828. The Commissioners also noted a 'singular informality' in Mercer's licence which had failed to specify the number of patients of each sex or to distinguish between them when describing the accommodation. This seems to demonstrate a lack of enthusiasm for complying with the certain aspects of the regulations. There was evidence too of a closer individual examination of the patients as with Mr Kiddle whom they found 'in a very imbecile and lost state of mind and not fit to take care of himself'.

Alongside the Lunacy Commissioners the Visitors continued their work of inspecting the asylum and had, since 1835 regularly comprised three Justices of the Peace including Lord Stavordale (Fox-Strangways), Lord

Digby and Sir William Oglander of Parnham House. In addition physicians Samuel Bradley of Yeovil attended for 13 years and William Shorland for 16 years. Their fee remained at £3 3s. 3d. for each visit as was the case for the Clerk of the Peace who attended and recorded details. Both the local Justices and Commissioners appeared to follow their own agenda without interaction as inspections of the asylum took place sometimes in the same month (June 1844, October 1848 and March 1853). No visits were made by the Lunacy Commissioners in 1849 and 1850.

Inspections continued to be recorded for the court without incident until May 1856 when a report worthy of commissioners Samuel Gaskell and Robert Lutwidge was made in respect of a cottage situated at the rear of the premises. They observed that it had been brought into use but thought it unfit for occupation as it was 'dilapidated gloomy and destitute of furniture'. The commissioners continued to report a lack of a proper bed and washing facilities and considered that the gentleman living there, who had been placed twice in restraint, should be removed to another asylum and were of the opinion that any future patients should be 'of a quiet and orderly class'. They stated that the cottage should be excluded from the licence. No plan of the premises was forthcoming when they requested it and the case book entries were 'still very vague and insufficient'.

The Commissioners continued to take an interest in patient comforts. In March 1858, they reported that there was a lack of bedding for one of the male patients which was 'insufficient for season'. Attention was brought to the courts of the failure, once again, to complete the case book correctly. Clearly they were having some difficulty in getting the Mercers to take action on issues made known.

In 1844 the report presented to Parliament by the Earl of Shaftesbury noted the twin aspects of Halstock asylum that would be a running theme for the next few years. The proprietor and staff were generally kindly and looked after their patients, but that the physical accommodation was not up to scratch.

> At Halstock the proprietor seems kindly disposed towards his patients; but the rooms occupied by two of them have been reported upon at our different visits as defective in every respect. At the last visit they were described as low, dirty, and without any furniture except a wooden bedstead.[310]

310 *Report of the Metropolitan Commissioners in Lunacy to the Lord Chancellor,* 1844.

In early December, 1844, a fire occurred which destroyed a large part of the building. An overheated stove had resulted in the destruction of a substantial part of the building used by the more violent patients, no injuries had been sustained. The Visitor's reported that one male patient had escaped during the fire, but he was found to be with 'friends'. It is notable that displaced patients were accommodated by others in the parish following the fire and there does not appear to have been any adverse public reaction. Surprisingly the incident was not reported in the local press. If concerns had been raised in the wake of the fire, with patients locked in their rooms or to their beds, they were not recorded.

Information concerning the rebuild was not forthcoming. The Visitors noted that nothing had been settled between occupier and owner who was at that time John F. Pinney. Problems continued and ten months later John F. Pinney had died which put a further delay on any 'definitive arrangement' relating to its restoration being made. The immediate outcome, reported by the Visitors, was that Mercer intended to apply for a shorter six month licence at the next Sessions so he can 'suit himself' if necessary with other premises.

Some insight into the problems encountered in rebuilding the asylum can be found in a letter dated January 1846 from John Justinian Mercer to Mr T. Fooks, clerk to the Quarter Sessions. It relates to his usual correspondence with the owner of Portland House, Mr Pinney:

> I am almost afraid to send Mr Pinney the purpose of the minute of the Visitors as I once did and it had not the desired effect in hurrying him - you see by the reports that I was absent each time of the Visitors coming here, my being so was on purpose as I could not bear to meet them unless the building had been begun - I assure you ever since the Fire my situation has been anything but enviable not a room to myself by day and at night exposed to the noise of my unfortunate Patients, in fact I am almost unnerved - Believe me. [311]

It appears that Mercer had been regularly sending copies of the Visitors' reports to Mr Pinney; perhaps it was a contractual matter. When he wrote this letter John F. Pinney had died in the previous September, leaving his estate to his son William who was perhaps concerned with other matters and did not have the same strong association with the Mercer family that had been developed in the previous generations.

311   DHC, *Correspondence and Abstracts of Acts etc 'State of Halstock'* (Q/A/L/ Bundle 5, 1846).

Part of the house remained habitable despite the fire and delayed building works. The Visitors reported that it was very overcrowded with 14 patients. The Lunacy Commissioners also stated that should the outer wing not be 'speedily done' before the winter it could affect the asylum's licence renewal. In the midst of this difficult time a particular damning report was made by the Commissioner Edward Seymour in January 1846:

> I have gone over this asylum and seen the patients; it is one of the worst asylums I have ever seen and is in my opinion totally unfitted for the proper care and treatment of insane patients.

Lord Edward Seymour, a Liberal MP, was one of the six honorary commissioners who were appointed mainly as board members.[312] He is not known to have visited Halstock on previous occasions. Seymour was accompanied by his brother-in-law Richard Brinsley Sheridan of Frampton, a Justice of the Peace, High Sheriff of Dorset and M.P. for Shaftesbury. He was the grandson of his namesake, the playwright Richard Brinsley Sheridan and his sister Georgina Sheridan had married Lord Seymour.[313] Sheridan having some previous experience of visiting the asylum chose to add to the critical report saying that it was:

> in its usual dilapidated condition ... John Hood appeared in an excited state taking exercise in a dirty yard quite unfit for an insane patient ... Mr John Withye has been in an excited state for the last two weeks' [and had been locked in his bedroom].

He also noted that the entry made in the care book was not satisfactory. Mercer was said to be absent at the time, although he would have seen the report as it was annotated with 'True Copy, Mercer'. Neither Seymour or Sheridan are named as 'Visitors' for Halstock in the Quarter Sessions records, nor is their report recorded in the Quarter Session register; nor was any record made of further visits.[314]

The state of the asylum had not improved by the June of 1846 when it was described by Lunacy Commissioners, Mylne and Turner:, in the next report:

312   Fisher 'Seymour Edward Adolphus, Lord Seymour', *History of Parliament*
313   *Burke's Landed Gentry*, 'Richard Sheridan'.
314   DHC, Q/A/L/Private 3, Bundle 9.

the patients of all classes and of both sexes are crowded into the dwelling house occupied by the proprietors family, the construction and arrangement of which are exceedingly defective.......If Mr Mercer was to apply for a licence very probably be refused.[315]

The rebuild took almost three years. In June 1847, the Commissioners, Proctor and Prichard, noted that the new buildings were completed and that Mr Mercer intended to include them with the other premises in his next licence application. The Visitors stated that the new rooms consisted of two sitting rooms and two bedrooms each accommodating three patients and one patient in the remaining bedroom. The garretts appear to still be in use as they were noted as being 'perfectly free from any offensive smell'. At a visit made in October 1847 the sizes of the rooms were noted. The smallest room was a bedroom at 14' x 10' with two other rooms measuring 16' x 14'. The next visiting Commissioners, Mylne and Turner, reported with some reservation in October 1847 that the property had been improved. The accommodation was for six patients and their attendant, but the lack of internal communication between it and the main buildings was regretted. They also disapproved of the low bedroom ceilings which hampered room space and ventilation.

In September 1848 it was reported the 'asylum suffered great loss in death of Mr Mercer of typhus fever', nobody else in the house was affected.

Business resumed. The court recorded that Harriet Mercer was 'anxious to retain management of asylum' and the Visitors were shown letters from friends and relatives expressing satisfaction with care; they wished her to continue. Harriet Mercer wrote to the Quarter Sessions separately with news of her husband's death. A copy of her letter was recorded in their minutes:

> Mrs J. J. Mercer is exceedingly sorry to announce the decease of her late husband Mr John Justinian Mercer Wednesday the 20 inst. of typhoid fever any inaccuracies she may have made in the accompanying papers she hopes will be excused.[316]

Barely a month later, in October 1848, another event was reported which was unlikely to have been viewed favourably in respect of renewing her licence. One of the married female patients had given birth (see the case

315   Ibid..
316   DHC, Q/A/L/Private.

study for Amelia Lindquist). This incident may have instigated a change of direction for the asylum as just 12 months later in October 1849, and without prior warning to the court, the Visitors found the asylum at Portland House closed; it was their third visit that year. Of the five patients one male patient had been taken to the Somerset County asylum in Wells which had opened earlier the same year, another removed, and the remaining three patients moved into a different property. Harriet Mercer had been refused a licence for five patients a month earlier 'on the ground (sic) of irregularity' and she had initially declined to reapply.[317] Her next application for a licence was refused again in January 1850 'on account of informality'.[318] The 'irregularity' of 1849 was chiefly Harriett Mercer's failure to keep a proper record detailing the unaccountable birth of a child in the asylum. This was the first and only time any such refusal for a licence was recorded for Halstock.

Confirmation of Harriet Mercer's move from Portland House and disposal of her deceased husband's equipment was recorded in the following newspaper advertisement:

Auction - 26 September 1849 - 'All the Neat and Valuable HOUSEHOLD FURNITURE and other effects, the property of Mrs Mercer who is leaving her residence......lists all contents including 12 feather beds, mattresses, washing stands, night commodes, towel horses, piano, easy chairs, kitchen requisites........' Also an Excellent stock of Medicine and complete Fittings-up of a respectable Surgery with many very valuable Surgical Instruments, and Books etc......' [319]

Harriet moved to another property in Halstock, described variously as 'House and Orchard', with her three remaining patients.[320] The property, by this time, had been owned by the Mercer family for 25 or more years and, according to the Visitor's report, it had previously been licenced. Her move seems to have been pragmatic; the house needed attention which was a constant financial burden, there had been difficulties with the landlord following the fire, the death of her husband had greatly reduced the asylum's ability to manage troublesome patients and there had been significant criticism from visiting officials. The old house was simply too large for her needs.

317   DHC, Q/S/M1/18, f.246.
318   Ibid., f.261.
319   *Sherborne Mercury,* 22 September 1849.
320   DHC, PE-HAL/CW/1/2.

HALSTOCK ASYLUM, DORSET.

TO BE SOLD BY AUCTION,
By MR. POOLE,

On the Premises, on WEDNESDAY the 26th of SEPTEMBER, 1849, and following day;

ALL the Neat and Valuable HOUSEHOLD FURNI-
TURE and other Effects, the property of Mrs.
MERCER, who is leaving her residence: comprising handsome mahogany four-post, field, and other bedsteads, with
moreen, chintz, and other furniture, window curtains, 12
excellent feather beds, bolsters and pillows, mattresses,
bed and table linen, mahogany and other chests of drawers, dressing tables, washing stands, night commodes,
towel horses, carpets and hearth-rugs, mahogany dining
and other tables, chairs, pier and dressing glasses, pianoforte, sofas, easy chairs, prints, books, fenders, fire-irons,
coal scuttles, kitchen requisites, kitchen range, handsome
stove and other grates, washing and brewing utensils;
malt mill, furnace, and other effects too numerous to par-
ticularize.

Also, an Excellent Stock of Medicine, and complete
Fittings-up of a respectable Surgery, with many very
valuable Surgical Instruments, and Books, &c. ; a small
rick of excellent Meadow Hay, a capital Horse, 6 years
old, fifteen-and-half hands high, good for harness or saddle, 1 Side and 2 other very good Saddles.

The Sale will begin each day precisely at Eleven
o'Clock in the forenoon.

Hand-bills may be obtained at the QUIET WOMAN INN
in Halstock, or at the Offices of Mr. POOLE, Surveyor
Auctioneer, &c., Sherborne, Dorset.

Confirmation of Harriet Mercer leaving Portland house. Details of the forthcoming auction including 'an Excellent stock of Medicine and complete Fittings-up of a respectable Surgery'. Sherborne Mercury, 22 September 1849

Unfortunately Harriet's move did not immediately solve her problems. Upon their first visit in October 1849 the Visitors, John Goodden, George Harbin and Dr Shoreland, found that she was operating outside the legislation in retaining more than one patient in an unlicenced house. Harriet Mercer had been under the impression that her licence would remain in place until 17 November 1849. The problem was resolved by assuring the Visitors that two of her patients would be immediately taken away and cared for separately in the homes of two people. This pragmatic solution was accepted by the Visitors although it hardly seems to have been within the spirit of the legislation. It may also indicate the high regard for the Mercer family within the community that after all their difficulties she could still draw upon the goodwill of her friends and neighbours.

Harriet Mercer was not granted a licence until over a year later in December 1850, it was to run for just 10 months which meant she would need to seek a new licence at the following Michaelmas Quarter Sessions.[321] The new house was equipped with six bedrooms, three attics, a kitchen, a back kitchen and other useful offices. In the census of 1851 Harriet was recorded as 'Proprietress Private Asylum' aged 40, living with her aunt, by marriage, Betsy Mercer, then aged 80, and two young servants, one male and one female, both aged 19. The household was completed by four patients who were identified only by initials and described simply as 'Lunatic'. Harriet continued for a further seven years with general approval from the visiting authorities. Only once, following a visit in 1856 by the Commissioners, Proctor and Wilkes, was it suggested suggested that in their opinion the house could accommodate no more than three patients. This comment was at odds with the previous Commissioners visit only a few months earlier when they authorised the licence to cover eight patients.

In 1857 the court record reported that Mrs Mercer was absent from the asylum at a time of inspection and that the patients had been left in the 'care of a young girl who acts as a servant which we think is hardly sufficient'. Mrs Mercer apologised in a letter saying she never left the village without leaving a responsible person or her sister 'who is in all respects as myself'. She added that the servant was a 'very steady and highly respectable person'. The asylum's final year was 1858 during which time there was no indication that it might be on the verge of closing, the accounts show the annual licence fee was paid in 1857, unchanged at £15. At the final report in July 1858 the Commissioners in Lunacy, Campbell and Nairne, wrote:

321   DHC, Q/S/M/1/18, f.329.

Since our last visit on the 11th March one of the female patients who was there in the House has been discharged recovered; the other four Patients, viz, 2 males and 2 females are still here and we found them quiet and in fair bodily health today. It appears that there has been no restraint or seclusion employed, and that none had been under Medical treatment. The House is in good order and the bedding comfortable. We have no special remark to make as to the condition of any of the inmates who appear to be in their usual state, and who we understand have the same means of occupation and amusement as have before been reported.

There was no immediate crisis. Whatever reason Harriet Mercer had for closing the asylum at Halstock it was not the result of pressure from the authorities. She had overcome the difficulties of a decade earlier and the asylum was once again an orderly and well managed house. A notice was published in the local newspaper announcing the sale by auction of the 'whole of the neat and modern Household Furniture, Pianoforte, China, Glass, Ware, excellent Pony Carriage and Harness, Bridle and Saddle, and other valuable Effects'. Instructions had been received from Mrs Mercer, 'who is about to leave the neighbourhood'.[322]

The fate of the four patients was not recorded in the Quarter Sessions. In-house patient registers during this time were not kept and individuals were rarely referred to by name by the Visitors. Of the four, as had been recorded by initials only on the census of 1851, the singular possible match for 'W.C' is Revd William Clarke, aged 51. A widower, from Perris Hill ('Rosina Hill' in the census) in Somerset, he had been admitted to Halstock asylum by his father in 1841 and was said to be incurable. No further information about him is forthcoming nor can the other three other people be identified from the asylum patient registers. They are listed only as:

C.W. male, 50 years old, unmarried and from Yeovil, Somerset.
M.F. female, 40 years old, married and from Cheddington, Somerset.
H. G. W. male, 52 years old, unmarried and from Yeovil, Somerset.

Perhaps they remained with Harriet for some time as paying guests. Three years later Harriet, aged 54, and her son John Justinian, aged 19, were in Hammersmith, London. The 1861 census showed she was a 'Landed Proprietress' and he an 'Articled Clerk'. Another resident listed

322 *Western Flying Post, Yeovil,* October 1858.

at the same address was from Yeovil, Elizabeth Whitmarsh also a 'Landed Proprietress' aged 60 - a person by the same name was admitted to the asylum in 1843.

Harriet retained a presence in Halstock in her ownership of a house, garden, and orchard occupied by Charles Gooch in 1863, the rent being £18 16s.[323] Harriet returned to Dorset where her sudden death was recorded at Evershot, 10 miles from Halstock, on 26 February 1867 in the house of J Clapcott.[324] The National Probate Calendar discloses she left effects valued at under £450.

In her will of the same year Harriet left a number of interesting bequests.[325] In addition to her estate which she gave to her son John Justinian Robert Constantine Whitely Mercer she gave £10 a year to her former servant Harriet Day of Yeovil for her life and after her death Eliza Bengefield of Chilthorne Domer was to receive £5 a year. Following Eliza's decease £5

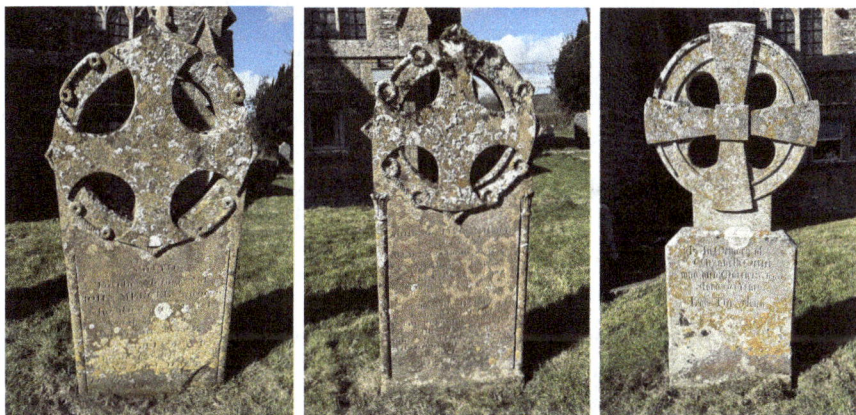

Mercer family gravestones of John Mercer, surgeon, aged 42 d.1818, John Justinian Mercer, surgeon, aged 34, d.1848, with Harriet Mercer, aged 66, d.1867, and Elizabeth Mercer, aged 90, d.1857, at Halstock parish church.

was to be given to Amelia Lindquist, the daughter of the patient who had become pregnant whilst in the asylum. The poor people of Halstock were given £3 a year to be spent on coal and distributed in the winter by her son, John Justinian. In 1871 he was aged 30, married and living in Burton Bradstock with three children. His occupation was given as 'Gentleman and

---

323   DHC, PE-HAL/CW/1/2.

324   *Sherborne Mercury* (12 March 1867).

325   DHC, NG-PB/1/8/26, *will of Harriett Walters Mercer,* (1867).

Landowner' and on his death in 1915, his effects were valued at the not inconsiderable sum of £21,266.[326]

Following the Lunacy Act of 1842 more importance was attached by the Visitors to the benefits of participating in the meagre activities on offer for the benefit of the patients and the Visitor's were expected to report on any noticeable effects. It appears that this was achieved by taking the time to question the patients and, whilst individual activities were not detailed, some understanding can be gained by the fact that in 1846 patients expressed the fact that they had 'much liberty'. This liberty was seen and noted on occasions when patients were found to be 'walking out' in the neighbourhood. After Harriet Mercer had moved the asylum the Lunacy Commissioners, Proctor and Hume, noted in 1851 that patients were able to exercise in the field adjoining the house owned by the proprietor. In 1857, it was observed that the gentlemen were 'free to take exercise' and that Miss Whitmarsh 'always goes to church when weather permits'.

Occasionally patients escaped. Amelia Lindquist's case including her escape is discussed in the case studies. Another patient who removed himself was John Withye junior, a widower and maltster from Sherborne, who was brought to the asylum by his father in September 1844, aged 44, and described in his assessment as 'curable'. His 'escape' was reported in December but it was discovered later that he had been staying with friends following the fire at the asylum; his return was noted in March 1845. Presumably he remained at the asylum for most or all of the rest of his life as, when he was buried in Sherborne aged 49 in 1848, his place of abode was initially given as Sherborne, but crossed out and replaced with Halstock. His death was not mentioned in the asylum register.

Understandably payment for patients, both pauper and private, may not have always been forthcoming. Sometimes the funds to support private patients were exhausted. An example of this can be seen in two letters sent to Mercer from Vining, a solicitor, in respect of Hannah Wilkins who was privately funded, in December 1846. The first stated that:

> it is not my intention to pay your bill in this matter, I will however write you in a few days on the subject, though I fear that my communication will not be satisfactory to you.

326 *John Justinian Robert Whitley Constantine Mercer,* (National Probate Calendar, Index of Wills and Administrations, 1858-1995)

The solicitor Mr Vining's letter to John J Mercer in February 1847 to explain that the funds for Mrs Wilkins were now exhausted and that the only hope of payment was directly from Mr Wilkins. DHC, D-FFO/29/11.

Transcript of second letter:

Sir, Had I any funds in my hands I would most readily remit you the amount over to you for Mrs Wilkins board etc., but I have none and am not in anyway responsible for it, and therefore cannot make you any remittance. I am satisfied now that her estate is exhausted and that your only means of getting paid is by application to Mr William Wilkins.[327]

The eventual outcome of this matter is not recorded. There must have been many other private patients in similar situations, such as Philip Keane whose fees were overdue in 1829. In other cases families may have found themselves unable to pay because of a change of circumstance in their business or personal affairs or complicated by inheritance disputes following

327 DHC, D-FFO/29/11.

a death. In these circumstances the once private patient might be removed from Halstock by their parish overseers if they became dependent upon the parish. This occurred in the case of Mary Spear who had been admitted as a private patient, said to be incurable, by her father in 1809. Twenty years later she was still listed in a letter from Alice Mercer to the Quarter Sessions amongst the private patients. However, in 1839 she was moved to Forston, aged 59 and now documented as a pauper patient, her fees chargeable to her home parish of Bere Regis.[328] This outcome for Mary was particularly well documented, but unlikely to have been an isolated case.

In some respects that the pauper patients represented a much lower financial risk to the asylum proprietors, funded as they were by their parish of origin and therefore less likely to abscond or default without the prospect of financial recovery.

From 1842 the Visitors were obliged to record the illness, general health and cause of death. Of the 270 people recorded as patients at Halstock throughout its history, around 36 identifiable deaths were recorded, although causes were not always described. Epilepsy was frequently mentioned as a cause of confinement for many; its symptoms feared and origins misunderstood. Elisha Pearce of Lyme Regis died from the condition in 1843 and it was noted as a cause of death in two further cases. Diarrhoea, also called 'internal inflammation' was a cause of death on two occasions and there was one from 'influenza. Another patient suffered a stroke and there was one suicide. The remainder appear to have died from age related conditions described by the Visitors as a 'general decay of nature'.

The Quarter Session records contained the final annual register, with details of named patients, in June 1844-1845. There were 15 in total, two of whom left in the Spring of 1845 and one who escaped in late 1844. From 1845 only the number of males and females were recorded, and patients were not named, apart from noting the death of John Hood in 1847. Other records were kept at the asylum, as a consequence of the 1845 Lunacy Act: case and patient books, a register of discharges and deaths, a medical journal and a register of admissions. All of which were inspected by the Visitors, none of which have survived.

Occasionally a combination of records from the Halstock asylum, the county criminal justice system and the county asylum allow a more complete set of biographical details to be established for some of the patients. While these individuals may not always have been representative their treatment and conditions are illustrative of the circumstances that may have been faced

328   DHC, NH-HH/CMR/4/32A/264.

by other inmates. In April 1845, John Justinian Mercer wrote to William Fooks, Clerk of the Peace, of Eliza Dowding's removal from Halstock to Forston the previous year. To inform the court was a legal requirement, but Mercer wrote an additional note which stated 'her state of health I consider to have been improved whilst she was here'. Perhaps Mercer was keen to convey his belief in the living conditions and treatments in his house, perhaps a concern too about her future care whilst not necessarily endorsing her removal.[329] Eliza Dowding's order paper drawn up on her admission to Forston in 1844 described her as suffering with a mental disability from birth, stated that she had 'always been of weak intellect', and noted that she might be violent and self destructive, and a 'dangerous idiot'.[330]

Transcript:
Asylum
Halstock April 21st 1845
Sir,
I am to aquaint you that Eliza Dowding of the Parish of Cerne Abbas was removed to Forston Asylum on the 18th day of April 1845 her state of health I consider to have been much improved whilst she was here.
I am Sir
Your obediant servant?
J Mercer
To Wm Fooks Esquire, Clerk of the Peace.

Before her spell at Halstock asylum Eliza had spent some time in the Cerne Union workhouse at the age of 21, where she was convicted for damaging workhouse clothes. A sentence of hard labour was given for one month. The records described Eliza as 4' 10¾", dark brown hair, blue eyes and fair complexion. Two years later in 1843, she was convicted of the same crime and received two months hard labour.[331] The following year in 1844, her sentence was two months hard labour for 'trespass; breaking [a] gate'.[332] Moving to Halstock, albeit briefly, and then to Forston provided her with some respite. Eliza was buried at Charminster in 1870 aged 52 with the note 'from asylum late of Cerne Abbas'.[333]

329   DHC, QAL/Private/3 1845.
330   DHC, NG-HH/CMR/4/32B/464.
331   DHC, NG-PR/1/D/2/3.
332   DHC, NG-PR/1/D/2/4.
333   DHC, PE-CMR/RE/4/2.

Letter from John Justinian Mercer to Forston asylum regarding the transfer of Eliza Dowding and stating that her health had improved during her stay, 1845. DHC, Q/A/L.

Eliza's situation was described again in the Forston medical journal which stated she 'has been here a long time and an 'imbecile from birth'. No change in any respect. Health good. No mental change. Is employed daily, quarrelsome, generally quiet'.[334] The patients' case register implied that there may be some hereditary condition in the family and described her mother as 'insane'.[335]

The patients at Halstock were from all backgrounds and ages. In 1852 David Elliott was the oldest admitted aged 80, he had been brought by Beaminster parish in a weak and emaciated state. He died a week later of erysipelas (a bacterial skin infection) after which the Visitors report an inquiry where they found 'every attention had been paid which his case required'. Had this situation occurred 50 years earlier it would have very likely passed without comment.

CRANBORNE

FOLLOWING THE LUNACY Act of 1842 inspections were made by a combination of local Justices of the Peace and members of the newly formed board of Metropolitan Commissioners. Together they visited the asylum on average six times a year between 1842 and 1848. This total of 36 visits was a considerable increase on the previous average of two a year and, although it was a legal requirement, this number might have been considered excessive in relation to the small number of patients. The Metropolitan Commissioners contributed twice yearly visits.

Between 1841 and 1848 William Symes was away from the asylum during six of the scheduled visits, sometimes at a distance of 30 miles or more, and sometimes he was away overnight. On one occasion an understandable concern was reported that only a boy of 16 and a female servant were left in charge at the property. Apparently in the event of an emergency help could be found at Symes' farm and from a woman who lived at the adjoining house who regularly assisted within the asylum. The Metropolitan Commissioners expressed concern that information required during their inspections could only be determined from the inmates and not from Symes himself. They requested that this was to be brought to the notice of the local Visiting Justices. The Commissioners were clearly unimpressed, he had failed to meet with them over their first three visits. However, not all

334   DHC, NG-HH/CMR/4/21/2.
335   DHC, NG-HH/CMR/4/13/1.

Symes' absences were reported with negativity as in June 1843 the Visitors found that he was absent together with three of his patients as he had taken them on an excursion.

Symes had failed to comply with several the administrative aspects of the 1828 Madhouse Act and this continued after 1842. He failed to produce the weekly medical journal which was requested in July 1843 and which all asylum keepers were obliged to maintain. Following the new legislation contained in the Lunacy Act of 1842 there was an increased level of reporting. In the October of that year the Metropolitan Commissioners, Proctor and Hawkins, made their inaugural visit. They observed that no patient was under mechanical restraint, discussed at length the resident with epilepsy, and noted the record keeping in both areas. The asylum was described as being clean and comfortable and the only negative element of their assessment was the absence of William Symes.

In October 1843 the Metropolitan Commissioners, John Hancock and Thomas Turner, advised the court that no patients were under constant restraint, although occasionally this was necessary overnight in respect of one male and one female patient. They also took exception to the fact that two gentlemen were sharing a bedroom. Further problems were encountered during their visit when a ceiling collapsed in one of the bedrooms which was said to be in a deplorable condition. For the first time the house was described as feeling damp and on such a rainy day the sitting room required the warmth of a fire, but it was a matter of some concern that 'no-one was mature enough to light one'. Their report was not entirely critical, describing the dinner as 'good and abundant', and noting that the patients engaged in the usual amusements of reading, writing and sewing. Returning to the negative aspects of their visit they once again reported that no medical book was produced. Nevertheless, the licence was renewed for another year.[336]

The problems found relating to sleeping arrangements were said to be rectified by March 1844 when apart from the two sisters sharing a bedroom all the other patients had rooms of their own. Two years later the subject was revisited when it was reported that the three best bedrooms on the first floor were all unused whilst the garrett rooms were occupied by the Blandford sisters and Mr Dale. No reason was given in respect of this arrangement nor were any observations made as to which rooms were occupied by the proprietor and other employees.

Reports made by the local Visitors and those of the Metropolitan Commissioners often differed both in content and length. In August 1842

336 DHC, Q/S/M/1/17 f. 285.

Section from Cranborne register transcribed for the Quarter Sessions for the year June 1843 to 1844. The eight patients, all private, show an equal number of men and women with four from within the county and the remainder from further afield. Their conditions varied with three said to be incurable, one relieved and one Jane Lanning said to be 'very much relieved'. Another, Fanny Gilbert, had been discharged in May 1844. DHC, Q/A/L.

the Visitors made a report quite different in content to that made by the Commissioners. They noted the attendance of church service and little else save the recognition that the iron bars had been put in place. One month later, in the following July, the Metropolitan Commissioners, Southey and Lutwidge, visited the asylum. Symes was absent and could not be questioned about the conditions. So, they offered an extensive report based entirely on their own observations of the general state of the house. Although it was ventilated properly, they stated that the sleeping areas were in a bad condition and that repairs were needed. Attention was brought to the daily activities of the three male and three female patients noting that one male was out walking and another two were reading, two were assisting in the kitchen, and the last was 'incapable of exertion of any kind'. Returning later in the same month the Visitors did no more than cover the usual basic information relating to cleanliness and clergy visits.

The report relates the inspection made by the three official Visitors to Cranborne asylum in May 1843. The content reflects the high level of attention placed on religious activities within the house. DHC, Q/A/L.

A full report was made in March 1844 when the Visitors, fulfilling their obligations to look at patient numbers and situations, stated that they found a Frances Gilbert at dinner with the servants in the kitchen. Gilbert, recently arrived on the 19th of the same month, had not been certified as insane nor was her name on the register. The asylum was in danger of over subscription, but assurances were made that John Ferris, who was away at the time on a visit, was about to leave and that this would bring the patient numbers back down to the six for which it was licenced. Thomas Edward, an employee of eight years, was said to be competent in the management of patients. The medical journal was produced for the first time and it was noted that two bedrooms had been papered and whitewashed.

The asylum received two visits from Anthony Ashley-Cooper in 1844 and 1845; he signed himself as 'Shaftesbury' in the Quarter Sessions records although he did not become the 7th Earl of Shaftesbury until 1851. He attended with the regular visitor Richard Brouncker and short reports of his visits were made for the court. Together they had inspected the apartments of all the patients and found them clean, in good order and in all respects well arranged. Only one patient was at home during the visit and he appeared to be in good health. They concluded that they had every reason to believe that this establishment was well managed.

In his capacity as one of the visiting Justices the Earl of Shaftesbury reported to the Quarter Sessions court on the conditions found at Cranborne asylum in October 1844.

Out of the ordinary incidents reported to the court were few and therefore they stand out in the records. In 1847 the Visitors found a male patient, aged 61, who can be identified from the admittance documents as Revd Edward Lloyd, with other patients in the parlour clothed in a 'straight waistcoat', a form of straight jacket. The record stated:

we do not think patients in the excited state in which we found him and using such language as he did, should be kept in the presence of others who are not violent and whose feelings may be injuriously affected by witnessing violence and hearing such language.

They continued that they did not believe that the asylum offered suitable accommodation for violent and abusive patients and that Mr Symes should confine himself to patients who were likely to be of a more peaceful nature. The Visitors expressed concern that the feelings of the others would be 'injuriously affected' and that they could not recommend the asylum had the equipment, accommodation of staff suitable for such cases. The Commissioners in the following month, reported the same patient in bed in a 'straight waistcoat'. No further comment on the matter was made. This situation must have upset the status quo previously afforded within the asylum. Having experienced the objections of his neighbours when he established the asylum Symes must have been mindful of his neighbours.

His asylum might be at risk if they were disturbed by a violent, loud or aggressive patient wandering at large in the town.

Revd Edward Lloyd had been admitted on 29 September 1847 by his wife. He was from Jersey and had been a patient at the large asylum at Laverstock in Wiltshire. His first attack of some form of mental disturbance had occurred 15 years earlier at the age of 46. Mr Symes wrote that he was violent, abusive and mischievous. The Commissioners reported that he was unfit to be associated with the rest of the patients and 'are glad that Symes had attended to their suggestions and put him in a room by himself'. Less than two years later his burial was recorded in the Cranborne parish records in 1849, aged 63, without mentioning that he had been a patient in the asylum.[337]

The Justices of the Peace reported that the situation had become more peaceful a few weeks later. In their longest report to date, made in January 1848. It was said that all of the patients were in a good state of health except one girl who was in bed, but only 'slightly indisposed'. Reference was made to a male patient, unnamed, but presumably the same Revd Edward Lloyd, who was now tranquil which made the use of the straight waistcoat or cuff restraint unnecessary. The state of one of the beds required immediate attention from Mr Symes, the Visitors expressed hope that there would be 'no reason to animadvert (make the same criticism) on the want of it again'.

There were concerns expressed relating to hygiene again in March 1848 when the Justices of the Peace reported that the 'sacking of the bed is offensive in the extreme' and recommended that the pan be cleaned with lime and that the sacking of bed be changed. They continued 'that if some means were not adopted to effect the purifying of this room then they would need to take the case into serious consideration'. Symes was again absent and the patients were under the charge of a male employee who had been employed by Symes for nearly 12 years. They had found a patient with bruising below the eye and a cut on his finger who said the injuries were from 'bad usage'. The man servant added that the patient had forcibly struck a box containing knives, but that he had no knowledge of how the bruise had been received. The Visitors reported the same patient had become violent and needed to be taken upstairs by two men, but, and more importantly it seems, no incidence of violence had been noted in the medical journal or the weekly report.

By the end of 1848 there had been no reports of restraint, no medical treatment and only one snap restraint at night. The patient numbers had

337   DHC, PE-CRA/RE/4/3.

Report made to the Quarter Sessions in September 1847 by two Visiting Justices and a surgeon. It details of the use of a 'straight waistcoat' to restrain a patient at Cranborne asylum. The Visitors suggested that William Symes should accept only patients without violent characteristics in future. DHC, Q/A/L.

fluctuated and there had been eight patients for a short period, but by the time of the report there were five, which was within the limits of the licence. The last report made by Henry Sturt and John Rowe in December stated conditions were much the same.

One patient who was not listed in the court register was Elizabeth Green whose details, albeit brief, were recorded in a bundle of small documents annexed to the Quarter Sessions records. She had been admitted in December 1846, said to be from Blandford and removed after a short time in June 1847 by Revd C. Green, when she 'having become quite well has returned to her friends'. In 1841 she had been living with the Green family and was then aged 35. She shared the house with Charles Green, her brother perhaps, who was the head of the family, a schoolmaster and clerk, aged 30, and his wife and children. Elizabeth suffered from depression and self destruction and died and was buried at Cranborne aged 44 in December 1848; cause of death was not recorded. The terms 'depression' and 'self destruction' were rarely used in the asylum records at this time, the preferred terms being 'melancholia' and 'suicidal', so perhaps the choice of language in Elizabeth's case highlighted particular concerns or an extreme condition, or perhaps a new understanding.[338]

Of the other 18 patients known to have spent time in Cranborne asylum one was said to be cured in under two years (Foss), three were relieved and discharged (Lanning, Pond and Gilbert) two were considered to be incurable and removed by members of their families (Beale, Simmonds), one, a child, was said to be an 'idiot' and was eventually transferred to a workhouse (Nation), one recovered (Hallett), one with no further information (Corbin) and three patients who had died during their incarceration (Smith, Lloyd, Ferris). Following the closure of the asylum the remaining six patients said to be 'not cured' were Frederick Dale, James Almond, the Blandford sisters, Thomas Parr Henning and Jane Oakley all of whom moved with William Symes to become patients at the Grove Asylum, in Nursling, Hampshire.[339]

Some details can be established on the patients who left with Symes. The stories of the Blandford sisters (discussed above) and Thomas Parr Henning reveal that those with sufficient capital to support themselves might live reasonably comfortable lives despite their conditions. Thomas Parr Henning was baptised in August 1817 to Thomas Henning and Mary (nee Parr) in Alton Pancras.[340] His admission paper notes that he had trained as attorney but never practiced. He was admitted by his aunt Harriet of Piddletrenthide on 7 June 1847, and was said to be incurable, violent at times and with a suicidal tendency.[341] In October 1847 the Visitors said that they had a long interview with him, at his request, and found him 'evidently in a very imbecile state of mind also subject to delusions'. When Cranborne

338   DHC, Q/A/L/Private/3.
339   TNA, MH 94/8.
340   DHC, PE-ALP/RE/2/1.
341   TNA, MH 94/7.

closed he accompanied William Symes to Grove Place asylum, but was removed from there in January 1855.[342] The same month saw Henning admitted to Westbrook House in Alton, Hampshire, a small private asylum for 30 people, only to be discharged ;'not improved' nine months later in September 1855.[343] Following his stay at Cranborne, Grove Place and briefly at Westbrook House asylums he returned to his family and was living, aged 43, with his mother, brother and two servants in Hampreston in 1861. The Henning family were wealthy and able to support themselves from investments and property. Ten years later the census listed him, his mother and brother in Sidmouth and by 1881, he was married and living in St Thomas, Exeter, where he was described in the census as a 'solicitor not in practice'.[344] He died in 1895, aged 77.

The final years of the Cranborne asylum saw little improvement in record keeping which remained a major concern for the authorities. William Symes was negligent in his legal responsibilities to the Quarter Sessions which he endeavoured, in part, to mitigate in a letter of explanation in May 1843. To Mr Fooks, Clerk of the Peace he wrote:

> I took a nephew to reside with me and assist me some months since and desired him to copy and send to you the order and certificates for the admission of Mr J Pond into my house, I did not know till I received Mr Sherring's note that he had done it and also the notice of the discharge of Jane Oakley and perhaps he did not send that. I shall therefore sent the necessary documents which I hope will not prove any inconvenience to you. I sent the young man away two months since for many acts of deception and falsehood and will be particularly careful in future to send every document required.[345]

If indeed Symes had been let down by his relation and employee he might have had the opportunity to remedy the situation. It appears to have been his intention to do so.

In another letter sent to Fooks in July 1844 Symes sought to offer some mitigation for his continuing failure to supply the correct paperwork: 'I have sent copies of reports, certificates etc. from register in case I should have neglected to have sent any The London Commissioners were here yesterday.

342   DHC, Q/A/L/Private/3.

343   TNA, MH 94/7.

344   *Census*, 1881.

345   DHC, Q/A/L/Private/3.

I have sent a copy of their report'. He continued that his five patients were Mr Dale, Mr Almond, the Blandford sisters and Jane Oakley. Jane Lanning, John Ferris, Fanny Gilbert and James Pond had all been discharged over the past six months and went on to explain that one of the visiting magistrates had borrowed his copies of the Acts of Parliament and therefore he had been unable to refer to the stipulations within them.

In September 1845 Symes wrote again to Mr Fooks with a copy of his report and a notice of application to renew his licence, stating that he was happy to make corrections if it contained any errors. The following month he wrote to Fooks again stating that he proposed

> to receive into such house four males and four females. And I further give you notice that I have the whole estate and interest in the aforesaid house and premises and that I propose to reside therein myself'.[346]

From the court records it seemed that Mr Symes rarely, if ever, achieved a licence for this number of patients.

Confusion and errors continued as the failure to maintain accurate records continued to exasperate the court officials. In at least one instance, relating to the attendance of the medical surgeon John Rowe in October 1845, it does not appear that Symes was found to have been at fault. Rowe stated:

> Not being able to find the account of which I sent you a copy last year I applied to Mr Symes to request him to send me an extract from the Visitors book which I now send, but there were other attendances, indeed it appears by Mr Symes' note that I made regulations which does not appear in the Visitors book. When you sent me the bill from Mr Symes for me to negotiate £12 10s. od. you observed there was more due to me but did not mention the sum - I shall leave it entirely with yourself I shall be satisfied with what you may think proper My attendance at the asylum has usually been by request of some one of the visiting magistrates, I shall feel obliged by your instruction as to my attendance for making the oath according to the new regulations as I have not yet been appraised of any meeting about to take place - I had never any instructions as the periods of visiting the asylum, 9 Oct 1845.[347]

346   Ibid.
347   Ibid.

Symes stated that he had made a record of the visits made by Rowe from the signatures in the Visitors book, but there had been at least six occasions between 1831 and 1844 where it appeared that Rowe had neglected to record his calls in the book. Symes was ultimately responsible to ensure that the records of his asylum were maintained correctly, but he was not always helped by his staff or the visiting officials.

MR. W. FURBER, without reserve, (by order of William Symes, esq., who is removing, having purchased Grove Place Lunatic Asylum, with all the Furniture and Effects), on the premises at Cranbourne, in the county of Dorset, on Wednesday, April 25, 1849, and following days, at 12 o'clock precisely, on account of the number of Lots. The whole of the FURNITURE, CHINA, GLASS, LINEN and EFFECTS of his residence, comprising 16 four-post, tent, French and iron bedsteads, 16 excellent feather beds and bolsters, 32 pillows, 20 mattresses, 30 pair of blankets, mahogany and painted wash-stands, dressing tables, chests of drawers, wardrobes, dressing glasses, sets of mahogany painted and stained chairs, Brussels and other carpets, easy chairs, sofas, couches, chimney glasses in gilt frames, sets of mahogany dining tables, four 8 day clocks, hall lamps, loo and card tables and side tables, secretary bookcase, two excellent piano-fortes, fenders and fire irons, a 20-gallon, copper, and a large quantity of kitchen requisites, china glass, &c., garden rollers, and tools, a chemist's still complete, bottles and cases, and a large quantity of excellent linen in sheets, table cloths, towels, &c., &c.

Also, at Penny's Farm, Cranbourne, on Monday, April 30th, at 12 o'clock, the remaining portion of FARMING STOCK, comprising four excellent cart horses, pair of black ponies (under duty), a splendid bay mare (warranted sound), a thorough good hunter, 6 years old, well known to the hunts in the neighbourhood, cow and calf, heifer in calf, phæton for one or two horses, with shifting head, four waggons, dung pot, light cart, spring pony cart, two strong gigs, phæton, set of brass mounted gig harness, set of pony ditto, 12 sets of cart harness, two side saddles, two iron rollers, drags, two pair of harrows, three ploughs, winnowing tackle, Amesbury heaver complete, four sets of plough harness, bean mill, turnip cutter (Gardener), wooden roller, scarifier, turnip hoe, wheelbarrow, an excellent 3-horse thrashing machine, stump of hay, four loads of good Ash Timber, with sundry useful articles.

The auction notice for the sale in 1849 of the contents of Cranborne asylum. Farm stock, implements, a variety of wagons and horses are listed. The inclusion of a chemist's still is the only item which could be used in a medical surgery. All other surgical equipment presumably stayed with William Symes. Hampshire Advertiser, 14 April 1849.

Despite his troubles Symes continued to be granted licences at the Michaelmas Quarter Sessions through until 1848 when his final licence was granted for three months only.[348] He left Cranborne asylum sometime in

348   DHC, Q/S/M/1/18, October 1848, f.173.

1849. A newspaper published a notice of an auction for the contents of both the asylum and Pennys Farm in the April of that year.[349]

William Symes left Cranborne and moved to Grove Place at Nursling, near Southampton, which had been adapted as a private lunatic asylum in 1813. He had no previous association with the asylum which accepted pauper patients as well as private patients. The asylum at Grove Place was amongst nine provincial houses named in the 1844 Report published by the Metropolitan Commissioners which justified 'almost unqualified censure'.[350] Nonetheless, he purchased the property with the appropriately named Isaac Pothecary as a part of Southwells Manor in 1849 for £5000.[351] The mortgage sum raised on the security of the premises themselves, and an interest Isaac Pothecary had in the estate of his late father.

A notice was placed front page in a Hampshire newspaper in July 1849 stating that William Symes, surgeon, who had conducted a lunatic asylum at Cranborne had with Isaac Pothecary, also of Cranborne, bought the asylum at Grove Place, which had already been established for 35 years. They further stated that the asylum will be managed by them and they would live at the premises to give constant care and superintendence. To give additional public reassurance they would continue to employ the resident medical superintendent who had been the visiting inspector for the previous 20 years.[352]

Additional information was placed in a notice in the same newspaper in October 1849. Grove Place Asylum was described as being for the reception and care of persons afflicted with nervous and mental diseases. Advertising as widely as Symes and Pothecary were able, they explained that the founder Edward Middleton, esq., a medical doctor, had established the institution without regard to expense and intended it to be for higher, middle and lower classes of society. It had a lawn of over 50 acres and had at one time been a royal residence. The air was said to be salubrious, the views pleasing, and farm produce was available from the estate. Importantly it continued with being in 'perfect accordance with the present improved moral and medical principles' avoiding restraint and providing trustworthy attendants.[353] Symes' former assistant from Cranborne Thomas Edwards was listed in the 1851 census as one of the attendants, aged 33, along with the five

349   *Salisbury and Winchester Journal,* 7 April 1849.

350   Parry-Jones, *The Trade in Lunacy,* p. 253.

351   Southampton University, Broadlands archive, MS62/BR/161/1-19.

352   *Hampshire Independent,* 21 July 1849.

353   Ibid., 20 October 1849.

previously mentioned patients; Frederick Dale, the Blandford sisters, James Almond, and Jane Oakley. There was also an entry for a Thomas Humming which may have been misheard for Thomas Henning who it was understood had joined the others at Grove Place.

A short time later there was evidence of trouble looming published in the Hampshire Advertiser in August 1851, it was the result of two court cases. Isaac Pothecary and William Symes were found to be liable for debts incurred, for £48 6s. 3d. owing to Richard Hoskins and to Josiah George the younger for £5 15s. 6d.[354] Another case was heard by the same court in 1852 which related to a complaint to recover £35 7s. 3d. for work done upon the asylum, the debt and costs were to be paid in a week.[355] In 1853 evidence had been found by the Hampshire Visiting Justices of the Peace that a patient had been severely and cruelly treated at Grove asylum and and recommended that the licence be revoked.[356] By 1855 they both William Symes and Isaac Pothecary were declared bankrupts. When the case was reported in the local newspapers they were referred to as boarding house keepers.[357] William Symes died in 1855 aged 68 and was returned to Cranborne for burial. His place of abode was given as Grove Place.[358] A year later a newspaper reported in 1856 more details about the bankruptcy of Pothecary and Symes; it stated that Symes had died insane.[359]

Hampshire County Asylum was built on land at Knowle Farm near Fareham. Construction was completed in 1852 and in December the first patients were admitted from Grove Place, Fisherton House asylum and Carisbrooke asylum. The initial intake did not include any patients from Cranborne who had transferred to Grove Place; only those whose legal place of settlement was originally in the county of Hampshire.

Isaac Pothecary moved to Jersey where, together with his wife Eliza, they set up an asylum which was free from practising under English asylum legislation. Three patients from the early days of Symes's asylum in Cranborne were living with Pothecary at Bagatelle Retreat, Jersey, when the census was taken in 1861. One was Frederick Duodecimus Dale who had been at Cranborne in 1827, was said to be from St Andrews, London and

---

354 *Hampshire Advertiser*, 30 Aug 1851.

355 Ibid., 25 Sept 1852.

356 Parry-Jones, *The Trade in Lunacy*, p.247.

357 *Hampshire Chronicle*, 10 Feb 1855.

358 DHC, PE-CRA/RE/4/2.

359 *Morning Post*, 1 May 1856.

held the surgeon's qualification MRCS though noted as 'retired'; he was 72. The other two were Charlotte and Mary Ann Blandford, sisters, aged 62 and 58. All were described as 'boarders'. Ten years later all three were still with Pothecary, then aged 56, in his 'new' private institution with 15 'lodgers' known as Cranborne House, Grouville, Jersey.

FORSTON

THE SITUATION OVER overcrowding and lack of capacity at Forston was discussed at the Easter Sessions of 1844, plans were altered and estimates made but in order to make their case more clearly, the Visitors presented to the court the outcome of recent parish returns made in August 1843.[360] Pressure for places was evident - 35 'lunatics' and 91 'idiots' had not been placed in Forston and 20 of these remained in private asylums. Since the returns had been completed applications had been made for 32 potential patients, none of whom had been included on the returns lists. Places were found at Forston for 27 of these applicants. It was realised that the current patient provision fell short by some margin of the actual need, this was largely in consequence of inaccurate information having been presented by the parishes. The court was reminded that the asylum had been conceived at the outset to receive 60 patients, considered to be an adequate number for the county at the time.

In response, the asylum staff created places for some patients by turning rooms designed for staff into dormitories.[361] The attics in the superintendent's house were given up for the 'best class of patients', initially for three beds but necessity increased this number to six. A situation which was considered to be detrimental and could not continue. During this time the asylum had held 110 patients, 20 above what was said to provide proper accommodation. These conditions were unhealthy and likely to exacerbate the spread of disease; such concerns were presented to the court by the superintendent.

In 1844, the Metropolitan Commissioners made a particular reference to the value of outdoor labour as greatly encouraged by the medical superintendent.[362] This was likely to have been an essential part of daily life because space inside the property was cramped and uncomfortable. It

360   DHC, NG-HH/CMR/1/4/1.
361   Ibid.
362   DHC, NG-HH/CMR/1/4/1.

was also noted that extra land had been sought to extend the provision of activities and labour, but this had not yet been procured by the magistrates; a situation which was regretted. However, it is clear sufficient land was made available for the various farming activities in which many patients were engaged.

The merits of providing meaningful occupations to patients was consistently expressed by the medical superintendents, Dr Button and Dr Quick; the benefits could 'scarcely be over-rated'.[363] This would have been welcome news to the Quarter Session officials as aside from assisting in patient recovery, (even the 'imbecile and demented can be brought to dig and plant') the expenditure of the institution diminished. Dr Button said in his report of 1850 that improvements made amongst even the most troublesome patients was such that their friends on visiting would say ' if they can work here they can work at home'. Such was, he said, 'the popular ignorance' and misunderstanding of the continual effort made in respect of each patient.

Dr Button's report was followed by another glowing account came from the Commissioners in Lunacy, Brian Proctor and Samuel Gaskell.[364] They found the asylum 'remarkably clean' and ventilated and in 'excellent order'. Each area had been 'minutely examined', including beds which were turned over in the manner expected from

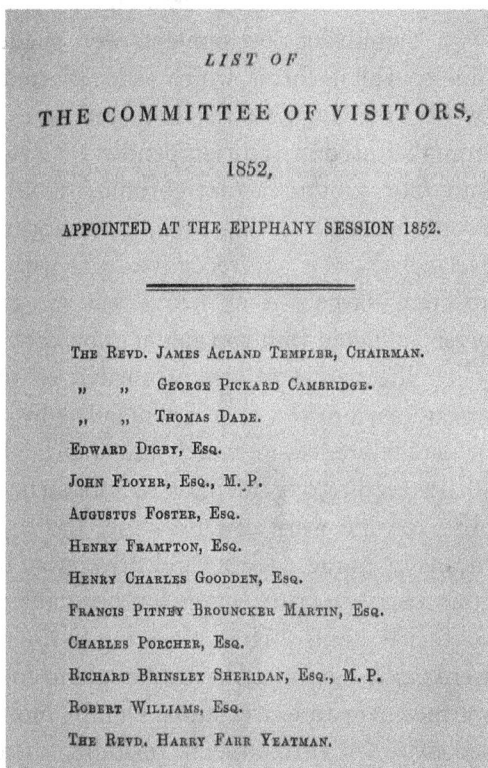

LIST OF

THE COMMITTEE OF VISITORS,

1852,

APPOINTED AT THE EPIPHANY SESSION 1852.

THE REVD. JAMES ACLAND TEMPLER, CHAIRMAN.

„ „ GEORGE PICKARD CAMBRIDGE.

„ „ THOMAS DADE.

EDWARD DIGBY, ESQ.

JOHN FLOYER, ESQ., M. P.

AUGUSTUS FOSTER, ESQ.

HENRY FRAMPTON, ESQ.

HENRY CHARLES GOODDEN, ESQ.

FRANCIS PITNEY BROUNCKER MARTIN, ESQ.

CHARLES PORCHER, ESQ.

RICHARD BRINSLEY SHERIDAN, ESQ., M. P.

ROBERT WILLIAMS, ESQ.

THE REVD. HARRY FARR YEATMAN.

Visitors appointed to the Forston committee in 1852. Of these Richard Brinsley Sheridan had visited Halstock in person, Henry Charles Goodden had connections to Halstock through his father Wyndham Goodden as had Edward St Vincent Digby, son of Sir Henry Digby. DHC, Q/A/L.

363   DHC, NG-HH/CMR/2/1/2.

364   DHC, NG-HH/CMR/1/1/1.

Mr Gaskell. They saw and tasted the 'ample' meal provided to the patients, which included beef and mutton, parsnips, carrots, bread and cheese, stating that it was all of very good quality. They extolled praise to Dr Button for his 'careful and judicious management'.

Two years later, in 1852, another positive report was made by Lunacy Commissioners Brian Procter and Thomas Turner 20 years after the asylum at Forston opened.[365] They found the asylum clean and 'free from offensive odours' and all the beds, none of which were loose straw beds, were found to be clean and comfortable. Patients' hands and faces were washed every day, bathed once a week and were well clothed and 'generally very neat'.

Significant developments were made to the identification of mental illness, in all its forms, which were reflected in terminology used at Forston. By 1852 the language used to record types of mental disorder had changed from that used in 1841 (Appendix 4).[366] Now forms of mania were divided into four groups: acute, chronic, remittent and puerperal. Of the 36 people admitted during 1852, the majority were acute, a total of 11 cases. Melancholia was still recognised but without detailed divisions, this time affecting six people. Dementia was recognised in seven people with one person afflicted with congenital imbecility.

The nature of any psychiatric or physical treatments at the three private asylums were never detailed by the Visitors or Commissioners beyond references to church attendance, physical exercise and occupations such as reading or gardening. At Forston in 1847 the Lunacy Commissioners observed the work of Dr Button, the superintendent who tried various means to 'purge' patients and drive away their illness.[367] Blood letting was commonly used particularly for those suffering from mania. Dr Button used counter irritants such as blistering to the nape of the neck. Cold poultices were applied to shaved heads thought to cool a heated brain, whilst feet were warmed to restore circulation. Opium, morphine and camphor were used as sedatives. Other treatments, including the use of drugs, were experimental and often discovered by accident and were tried and tested on patients in many asylums at the time.

Non invasive treatments such as the benefits of a good diet were also recognised by the Forston doctors (Appendix 3), indeed it was ranked highly amongst 'remedial measures'.[368] It was recognised that providing

365   DHC, NG-HH/CMR/2/1/2, p.12.

366   Ibid., p.17.

367   Rogers, *In the Course of Time*, p.19.

368   DHC, NG-HH/CMR/2/1/2, p.25.

wholesome and appealing meals, with attention to quality and quantity, contributed much to mental tranquillity and as a result the numbers of deaths diminished. Dr Button advised the Quarter Sessions in 1850 that levels of starvation was, in many cases, a viable cause of insanity. Life was prolonged with an extra allowance of food along with the addition of wine or brandy. To emphasise the importance of treatment by diet cases of patients were brought to the court. In one example, a man admitted in 1850, was in a skeletal condition. He had probably been kept too long either at home or in the workhouse and had 'passed into a state of dementia' and unlikely to recover; there were many more like him.[369]

Physical restraint mechanisms continued to be used although the Forston Visitors reported it less frequently as the years progressed. However, the practice remained for some. The exact form of restraint was seldom mentioned, except in 1841 when 'muffs' had been used to confine a patient's hands for a short time. This method, which appeared to be new, had prevented one patient from self harm, suicide even, the benefit of which had led to the patient being cured and discharged. Further methods of restraint used were heavy harnesses, ankle cuffs and belts with leather sleeves, each amounting to eight to ten pounds in weight.[370] Additionally there were metal handcuffs and padded leather cuffs which could be strapped to the body or the bed. By 1852 routine mechanical restraint had ceased at Forston, mostly due to the influences and new approaches brought by Samuel Tuke's 'moral treatment'. For those who were 'violent and maniacal' a treatment of seclusion was used to calm and tranquilize patients, such was reported by Commissioner James Mylne in October 1852.[371] He also noted that no 'instrumental coercion', in any form, was used.

In contrast to reports made by the local Justices and Lunacy Commissioners the annual reports provided to the Quarter Sessions by the onsite physicians reveal much about their understanding of mental health. This subject is largely missing from the reports made by medical men attending Dorset's private asylums, which were compiled for the purpose of recording specific information for the Quarter Sessions. In the early days Forston asylum benefitted from the appointment of two medical superintendents who had been trained at the highly regarded Hanwell asylum: Dr Quick and his successor Dr Button. Both brought their expertise to Dorset and set down from the beginning their visions for the future. This

369 Ibid., p.15.
370 Rogers, *In the Course of Time*, p.18
371 DHC, NG-HH/CMR/2/1/2, p.14

led to honest and comprehensive reports being presented to the Quarter Sessions; compiled by men who were in the vanguard of a rapidly emerging medical field.

Both Dr Quick and Dr Button extended their remits and wrote at length about their findings in all areas which were brought to the Quarter Session court every year.[372] Extensive attention was presented to describe disorders which coexisted with states of insanity. These were labelled separately as patients being subjected to either a physical or excited condition. Physical disorders were said to relate to paralysis, epilepsy, digestive problems and general poor health. Patients described as 'excited' predominantly suffered from 'intemperance' (unable to control behaviour with extreme moods); principally caused by distress. This condition, in turn, was attributed to the increase of beer-houses, the 'bane of the peasantry' and the temptation of drinking 'a fruitful source of so frightful a calamity'. [373]

Above all it seems that Dr Button held an appreciable understanding of mental health problems; reflected in his report of 1843. He explained that many potential sufferers did not necessarily display incoherence or become unable to display to some notable degree their former 'powers of mind'.[374] He recognised that mental disease had often prevailed long before these manifestations became obvious. Clearly, he knew that recognising the condition of insanity was far from straightforward but stressed that both medical and moral treatment would improve success rates if concerns were raised at the outset when witnessing 'inexplicable habits'.

This was to be his main theme, consistently raised in his annual reports to the Quarter Sessions, where he identified reasons behind this considerable difficulty. Much of the blame was laid at the door of parish officials in continuing their procrastination in conveying the insane poor to Forston.[375] The doctor's frustration in the matter is all too clear as he pointed out that keeping people in their homes, or in the workhouse, was not only a dismal situation for them but also made the asylum a place for just the 'hopeless and the dying'. This was not considered to be proper cases (and no doubt not proper use of public funds) for the asylum and despite calls for immediate investigation the situation remained. Clearly the question from the medics was why mental disease was 'so unaccountably and recklessly neglected' which inevitably resulted in little hope of recovery.

372   Ibid., pp.11-12.
373   Ibid., pp.11-12.
374   Ibid., p.16.
375   Ibid., p.18.

Fear of unknown future costs and unwarranted expense seems to have dominated decisions made by parish officials in sending people to the asylum.[376] In addition Dr Button indicated, in1844, that much time and 'useless expense' was spent determining to which parish the individual belonged. The situation was not helped by the current law which required numerous proofs of settlement often making difficulties for officials to unravel. Ultimately until the issue was resolved the unfortunate sufferer was prohibited from admittance to the asylum.

As the costs of sending people from their parishes to the asylum seemed to be the main reason for delay efforts were made, through the Justices, to better understand why it was better for all concerned to admit potential patients within a short while, ideally three months, after their first attack.[377] Dr Button was clear that if this process was duly followed it was likely that time in the asylum would be, on average, just four months. In monetary terms this amounted to £5 and therefore considered to be a less costly way to restore someone to reason.

There were also legal implications in delaying admission. In cases of neglect Dr Button's report of 1847 brought attention to the regulations of the County Asylums act, 1845, which imposed certain penalties on Relieving Officers and Overseers in not sending the insane poor to the asylum when the first episode of insanity occurred.[378] He went on to say that scarcely any of the parish officers who brought patients to the asylum were aware of the existence of such a law and were 'quite unconscious of the great responsibility attached to their office as well as the penalty to which they are liable'. The unwillingness to consider individuals insane was understandable, due in the most part, from concerns relating to the extra load placed upon parish rates but this, he said, was a short sighted policy.

An example of this situation was recorded for the court in 1850 which related to a case involving differences of opinion, and cover ups, amongst parish and union officials.[379] It concerned a woman, unnamed, who had been insane for a year and whose circumstance was reported on a number of occasions by the master of the union to the district relieving officer, the medical officer and the board of guardians. Nothing was resolved until it became too difficult to keep her any longer in the Union. She was in a bad state, her clothing required burning and her health was extremely poor. On

376   Ibid., pp 21-2.
377   Ibid., p.19.
378   Ibid., pp.27-8.
379   Ibid., p.17.

learning of her situation, particularly the fact that she had been insane for '*a year*', the Visitors instigated legal proceedings. Ultimately, yet unsurprising perhaps, the master of the union retracted statements previously made and that the blame was placed, by the relieving officer, on the clerk of the board of guardians.

Not all blame could be directed to the parish officials. Dr Button endeavoured to point out that family and friends of those afflicted also played a part in their, often extreme, reluctance to admit the existence of insanity amongst loved ones.[380] This, he said, applied to all classes of society and noted that this 'direful calamity probably affected all families in various degrees. Several cases were relayed to the court over the years demonstrating the outcome of late interventions; many patients did not survive.[381] However, amongst these there were success stories. One case described a labourer, aged 58, who had been insane for five weeks, it was his second attack and he was said to be profoundly melancholic and suicidal due to poverty and all its 'consequences'. The parish overseer had apparently known that he had been 'bad some weeks' but had not intervened until finding him in the river with a razor. At this point Dr Button conveyed his deep frustration on the situation when he said that the afflicted man 'was now considered bad enough'; for the asylum. Following his stay at Forston with primarily treated with a 'nutritious diet' he recovered and was discharged.

In other areas Dr Button sought to improve procedures and in 1850 he requested additional information to be recorded on a patient's admission paper.[382] He explained that the paper did not require causes of insanity to be made known, nor its duration, and that an account from the patient themselves could not, obviously, be relied upon. Even information gathered from relatives could be less than truthful and gaining an understanding of the patient's background was key to finding the best way forward. He continued with the statement, in contrast to common belief, that insanity rarely occurs suddenly and without previous symptoms in someone who displayed apparent health. More often than not signs of problems had preceded the first attack but passed unnoticed by others. Dr Button concluded that the most common early symptoms was a change in the person's character, with 'pain in the head' and 'pervigilium' (wakeful all night).

380   Ibid., p.9.
381   Ibid., p16.
382   Ibid., p.9.

E. S.   On the application for the admission of this patient, it was stated by the Relieving Officer, that she had been " insane only a week," in consequence of which, though at considerable inconvenience, the Asylum being full, she was admitted : on her arrival, however, it was at once discovered that she was labouring under that most certainly fatal of all the various forms of Insanity, General Paralysis—and presented an appearance of being little, if at all, removed from complete idiotcy.   Her speech was embarassed—her tongue tremulous—her gait unsteady.   She was extremely incoherent, her memory was lost, and she was subject to sudden accessions of maniacal excitement.   It was, moreover, stated, that she was *not* the subject of Epilepsy, within, however, a few hours after her admission, this representation was also found *not* to be correct.   She was seized with a violent and protracted epileptic attack.   She was subsequently visited by her parents, from whom it was ascertained, that she had been the subject of mental alienation for a period of *not less* than *nine* months;   she had left her situation where she had

Forston's medical superintendent brought various examples of the insane poor to the attention of the Quarter Sessions. The case of E.S. describes her admission to the asylum despite it being at full capacity. It also relates the confusion surrounding the diagnosis of epilepsy. DHC, NG-HH/CMR/2/1/2.

This led to acknowledging the importance of proper sleep.[383] It was also said that patients brought to the asylum in the early stages of illness would benefit from both a change of scene and the assistance of the 'judicious administration of a narcotic'. Many cases of insanity could be prevented by providing such treatment before the onset of 'mania'.

Generally, the records relating to Forston asylum were positive. Whilst it is unfortunate that private views of local officials and Commissioners who shared the task of visiting all Dorset asylums remain unknown, a sense of relief amongst all can be gathered from examining the surviving documents. Despite many problems there was a palpable positive determination to make it work and be properly accountable; much was made of its success in the local newspapers. And, importantly for the regular communities, nobody was now seen to be getting rich quick, making money out of the suffering and costing the earth to parishioners.

383   Ibid., p.11.

HERRISON

	Male.	Female.	Total.
Admitted since the opening of the Asylum in 1832	335	410	745
Discharged	160	191	351
Died ..	107	114	221
Escaped	—	1	1
In the Asylum on the 31st December, 1849 ..	67	88	155
Admitted since	23	28	51
Discharged, Recovered ..	15	13	28
Ditto, by desire of friends	0	2	2
Died ..	7	6	13
Remaining 31st December, 1850 ..	68	95	163
Patients Admitted, Discharged, and Died during the Quarter, ending 31st December, 1850.			
In the Asylum on the 30th September	71	91	162
Admitted since ..	6	7	13
Discharged	7	0	7
Died ..	1	3	4

Details of the insane poor confined at Forston as presented to the Quarter Sessions from 1832 to 1850. It provides numbers of those who had died and escaped. Importantly it shows of those admitted almost half had been discharged. DHC, NG-HH/CMR/2/1/2.

BESIDE THE DAY to day running of the asylum discussions were continuing in the background, over many months, as to how to resolve the overcrowding crisis at Forston.[384] Expansion was first considered at either land to the north or south of the existing property and, in 1856, detailed expenses were drawn up which looked closely at both scenarios. Apart from erecting new buildings both plans implicated changes to the area and landscape one of which involved altering the course of the river

384   DHC, NG-HH/CMR/1/1/1.

Cerne. Forston was able to accommodate 140 patients but due to pressure on places an extra 15 patients had been received. To meet the increased demand the new building, on which ever new site was secured, it was decided that provision for 140 additional patients was required. There was also a necessity to return 42 patients currently housed at Fisherton to Forston which would bring the total number of registered Dorset patients to 197. There were currently 155 patients at Forston which, with the 42 at Fisherton asylum, amounted to a total of 197 registered Dorset patients. The plan was to eventually provide places for 280, resulting in accommodation for approximately 83 'fresh patients'.

Mr Evans attended the meeting and produced two plans, one for building on Sturts land on the south side of the asylum and the other on Sheridans land on the north side of the asylum. Each plan to accommodate 140 additional patients.

Perhaps it was realised that any outcome from either of these plans would not (and could not) fulfil an uncertain brief. The data provided by the parishes and unions was unreliable and not always forthcoming. Out of this concern came the understanding that a new asylum on a different site was the only way forward. A site comprising 16 acres of land at Radipole Barracks was offered in 1858 but rejected as too small.[385] In the meantime Dr Finch's offer to take surplus patients at Fisherton at 13*s.* per week for two years was accepted, perhaps in recognition that any new build was going to take time.

The matter continued and in September 1858 the following possibilities were laid out to the Committee:[386]

1. Land called Herrison in Charminster offered by Mr Michael Miller.
2. Land in Allington (Bridport) offered by General Michel.
3. Pymore Farm (Bridport) of 40 acres, adjoining above offered by Mr Templer.
4. Carey, near Wareham offered by Mr Phippard.
5. Binnegar, near Wareham offered by Lord Eldon.

The Committee decided on the land at Herrison as the most suitable site and began the process of purchasing the 50 acres.[387] The County Surveyor said that the site 'could not be seen by a traveller on either the top

385   DHC, NG-HH/CMR/1/1/3.
386   DHC, NG-HH/CMR/1/1/3.
387   DHC, NG-HH/CMR/1/1/3.

or bottom roads to Sherborne'; the cost was said to be £5,710.[388] Plans were made for the old asylum at Forston to be sold at public auction.[389] However, it was found necessary to retain the premises at least for the construction period.

By 1863, John Floyer, chairman of the Committee, stated that the building at Herrison was almost ready, only the testing of the water and gas supply remained.[390] In December the asylum received its first occupiers, male patients from Forston, who were described as 'cheerful & tranquil & contented'. The newly erected church was able to seat 400 people. Patients were returned from Fisherton, the men housed at Herrison and all the women at Forston. No Dorset pauper lunatics were now at Fisherton where many had been accommodated over the previous decades. There were beds for over 320 patients; building costs were in excess of £27,000.[391] The head count at the end of 1863 amounted to 132 males and 147 females with four criminal lunatics remaining at Fisherton asylum.

By1864, the building at Herrison was ready for the female patients. Almost all were moved except those who needed the least supervision, some 24 patients, who were kept at the Forston site.[392]

At this time the Visitors were considering taking in private patients was well as paupers. They were to be charged a higher rate for maintenance, although they would be treated in the same way as the existing pauper patients. At a later meeting it was agreed that no more than 20 private of 'non-pauper' patients would be admitted to either Forston or Herrison, now referred to as the 'two County Asylums'. A public subscription raised £2,000 for treatment and the fee was set at 10s. per week for the admission of 20 non-pauper patients, whose selection was to be made by a Sub-Committee of the Visitors.

The asylum now had sufficient capacity to take patients from outside the County which in 1864 amounted to 84 males and 32 females. An additional group of patients were 'non pauper' who amounted to eight men and eight women. Altogether this put the number of patients at 439 accommodated in the buildings at Forston and Herrison. Non pauper patients from outside Dorset were not admitted. One criminal lunatic remained at Fisherton.

388   Rogers, *In the Course of Time*, p.21.

389   DHC, NG-HH/CMR/1/4/2.

390   Ibid.

391   Brown, *History of Dorset Hospitals*, p.174.

392   DHC, NG-HH/CMR/1/4/2.

The decision to accept non pauper patients from Dorset, and charge a higher fee, may have been designed in some way to off-set the extra costs incurred in building roads and a bridge for access to Herrison. Funding for this work was to have been generated by the sale of the old asylum at Forston. An extra £3,000 was now needed.[393] The failure to effect Forston's sale brought about the decision to further open admissions to non-pauper lunatic's from adjoining counties. At the time of the report, in 1864, only two female non-pauper patients had been admitted. One, originally from Weymouth, had been transferred from Fisherton and the other from Chardstock, then in Devon.

The take up of non-pauper or private patients either from Dorset or other counties to Forston was slow; 1865 saw the admittance of 15 patients, fairly evenly split between the sexes. Six patients were from outside the county and nine originally from within. Four patients without obvious links to Dorset had been transferred from other asylums whilst two women had been admitted from Somerset. The following year just seven private patients were admitted again with a variety of origins.

For the majority who were just above the pauper status the acceptance of non-pauper county patients to Herrison in 1864 was welcome, they were to be kept at Forston. Prior to this change in policy many people found themselves to be too poor for the private asylums, but a cost too great for the parishes to bear at the county asylum.[394] With the lack of other affordable provision people usually remained at home until they were considered to be paupers, their condition by this stage probably much weakened.

Effectively by 1864 there were two county asylums running side by side, with a distance of approximately one mile between them across tracks and fields; the distance by road was over two miles. The Superintendent had the unenviable task of overseeing the management of patients and staff in both buildings. This situation relied upon good and trustworthy staff. Their contribution was frequently highlighted in Visitor's reports earning a reputation for kind and careful treatment and 'orderly conduct'. Inevitably there were exceptions, one of which was relayed in a Visitor's report in 1864. The Superintendent had called into the female ward at dinner time unannounced and noticed the absence of beer on the table. Following a search he found the missing beer, meant for the patients, hidden in the nurses' cupboard. No acceptable explanation was forthcoming and the two

393   Ibid.

394   Brown, *History of Dorset Hospitals*, p.175.

nurses involved were dismissed. There must have been many more incidents which were not reported.

In 1865, the weekly maintenance fees for non-pauper patients from Dorset remained fixed at 10s. but higher at 12s. for those from outside the County. In another change, the Visitor's reserved the right to charge 14s. for those patients who were 'more than ordinarily expensive'.[395] The same year brought about another initiative. An agreement was made to receive 60 patients from Littlemore in Oxfordshire for four years, fees were set at 11s. 6d. and Poole were sending 13 patients at 11s. per week. A further 30 male patients were expected to arrive from Abergavenny asylum; arrangements were made to take on more staff. In 1866 it was reported that the main asylum was considered mostly full; Forston had room for 50.

Herrison together with Forston, which housed non pauper patients, continued through the century admitting more patients. By 1874 there were 481 patients and to relieve the overcrowding situation it was decreed that some of the harmless patients were removed to the workhouses of the Cerne, Bridport and Sherborne Unions.[396] Further building ensued at the Herrison site which made it possible to close Forston house in 1895; the building was sold in 1899. Growth continued and by 1900 there were 569 patients from Dorset and 39 from elsewhere. A further 99 private patients were accommodated from the poorer classes. Thirty years on the Mental Treatment Act of 1930 signalled a major change in recognising that mental health issues was an illness similar to any other, voluntary patients were now permitted and use of the term pauper lunatic was officially finished.[397]

Herrison closed in 1992.

ACCOMMODATION IN OTHER COUNTIES, 1832-1860.

INFORMATION GATHERED BY government committees and departments do not fully reflect the movement of pauper patients between asylums, sometimes at quite a distance. Dorset's new county asylum at Forston had relatively few beds when it opened in 1832 at just 60, increasing to 82 in 1835. Fisherton House, in Wiltshire, a private asylum was found to be accommodating 60 pauper patients out of a total availability of 100 in 1837. It was managed by Dr Finch who had been called upon for advice

395   DHC, NG-HH/CMR/1/4/2.
396   Brown, *History of Dorset Hospitals*, p.175.
397   Ibid., p.176.

when Forston was at the planning stage.[398] People were moved according to the availability of places across various asylums, regardless of their home parish and county. Particularly, patients were moved between Forston and Fisherton, as shown in both asylum's records.[399] The reasons for the transfers were not usually provided. However, in 1849 the Visitors reported the usual details of patient numbers but also included information that eight females had been removed to Dr Finch's asylum who were described as chronic lunatics. This might imply that Forston did not have the capacity to cope with this particular level of mental illness, or that the managers simply transferred the most difficult and time consuming patients to Fisherton.

Mary Hodder, a widow and pauper aged 58, was admitted to Halstock in early October 1840, sent by parish officials of St Peter's, Dorchester. The asylum's register showed she was discharged a few weeks later, on 24 October, not cured, and found herself in Forston the following year. Her situation was discussed by the Visitor's at the Easter meeting of 1841:[400]

Mrs Hodder, who for many years had resided in the Parish of All Saints, Dorchester being the wife of the Book Keeper to Russell's Waggon Office who was brought down to Dorchester by one of her sons, and having been put into a Fly [a type of carriage] was left in the street at the door of another son, then residing in the parish of St Peters but who stated his utter inability to receive his Mother in her State of Lunacy, she was therefore taken care of by the Parish Officer and ultimately conveyed to Forston.

Her case was revisited a few months later in October restating that Mary Hodder had been 'left by her son in a carriage in one of the streets at Dorchester' and subsequently taken under an order of two magistrates to a private asylum (Halstock) and subsequently to Forston.[401] It appears that despite much effort no evidence had been found relating to her legal place of settlement or home parish, so the County was to be responsible for her fees. Mary's order paper on entry to Forston added little information other than she had born five children, the cause of her insanity was unknown.[402] She was admitted to Fisherton 12 years later in June 1852 as part of a group

398   Parry-Jones, *The Trade in Lunacy*, p.47.
399   WSHC, A1/560/3A1/560/3.
400   DHC, NG-HH/CMR/1/4/1.
401   Ibid.
402   DHC, NG-HH/CMR/4/32A/299.

of 'chronic lunatics' and discharged after eleven years, not improved.[403] The date of her removal coincides with a set of patients who were returned to Dorset on the same day in December 1863, the new and enlarged asylum at Herrison was now able to provide suitable accommodation.

Other examples of this can be seen from examining the patient's register for Fisherton. Maria Davidge, aged 17, was initially admitted to the Dorset County asylum in 1850 and transferred to Fisherton a few months later. She was a pauper, of 'unsound mind' and was said to have been insane for three months. She was not considered to be dangerous, suicidal or epileptic. No record was made as to why she was moved out of the county, her home parish was Motcombe in Dorset.[404] Maria was one of a few female patients who were moved en bloc to Fisherton from Forston asylum in July 1850 including Clara Sanders, Mary Roper, Phoebe Barfoot, Mary Ann Joy and Mary Slade.

The relationship with Dr Finch and his asylums in Wiltshire continued for a number of years. His expertise was sought and visits were made to his establishments. The numbers of patients sent from Forston to Fisherton was recorded in the visiting committee books. In 1853, 49 Dorset patients had been transferred to Fisherton when 158 remained at Forston.[405] Contracts and financial settlements between the two asylums were made annually. In 1856 Dr Finch made an offer, which was accepted, to continue to take patients for the ensuing year. The fee per patient was 13s. This amount, almost double the regular maintenance fee accounted for patients at Forston, may reflect the fact that Fisherton took patients with more serious conditions, said to be 'chronic', and also criminal lunatics. One such lunatic, Louisa Adams, was sent to Fisherton on the order of the Secretary of State because Forston was full; her fees were 14s. 6d. per week, the bill amounted to £18 17s. for half a year and was payable by the county. With the overcrowding situation at Forston and the closure of the private asylums in Dorset sending patients to Fisherton may have been the only option available.

The costs to the parish remained the same whether a patient remained at Forston or was transferred elsewhere. The excess was paid by the County.[406]

Patients were returned from Fisherton to Forston when places became available. The Forston case register includes six patients admitted

403   WSHC, A1/560/3A1/560/3.

404   DHC, NG-HH/CMR/4/32B/737.

405   DHC, NG-HH/CMR/1/1/1.

406   Brown, *A History of Dorset Hospitals*, p.174.

from Fisherton in 1849 -1850.[407] William Baker of Piddletrenthide; Mary Grist of Cranborne; Mary Ann Rickett probably from Dorchester; William Stout of Wimborne; Martha Jenkins of Langton Matravers and Thomas Stone of Shaftesbury. Thomas was described as mischievous and noted to have received a blow to his head from a hammer. He had been in Forston before and had twice been admitted to Fisherton.[408]

When the replacement asylum buildings were constructed at Herrison patients were brought from Fisherton to the newly built and renamed Dorset county asylum which could now accommodate 300 patients.[409] In 1863 Georgina Cuff, aged 25 and originally from Blandford St Mary in Dorset, was returned from Fisherton and admitted to Herrison.[410]

Patients from other counties were also brought to Herrison: Catherine Dobbin, aged 28 and originally from Weymouth, was admitted in 1855 from the asylum in Belfast asylum,[411] Ellen Hyde, a school teacher aged 24, came from Kent County asylum in 1855, but this time no former connection with Dorset was noted.[412]

Others had spent time in multiple institutions: Ann Welstead had been admitted to Halstock aged 46, said to be from the parish, in January 1844. The register notes she was incurable and was discharged 30 July 1844 only to be admitted to Forston. Ann Wellstead, transposed to Willstead on her order paper, was a single woman, said to be aged 35 when she was admitted the same year from Halstock.[413] The document stated she was liable to injure others, destroy clothes and although she was also of a 'temperate' or calm disposition she was said to be of 'dirty propensity', was well educated with a melancholic temperament. A case register entry offered more detail stating she had once been a governess and had been incarcerated in both Bethlem and St Lukes asylums. The cause of her illness was said to be 'disappointed affection' and hereditary; her mother was said to be insane.[414]

Despite the opening of the county lunatic asylum provision for pauper lunatics was still being made in the the workhouse. In 1848-49 the

407 DHC, NG-HH/CMR/4/13/1.

408 DHC, NG-HH/CMR/4/32A/211, and NG-HH/CMR/4/32B/684.

409 Rogers, *In the course of time*, p.21.

410 DHC, NG-HH/CMR/4/32D/1401.

411 DHC, NG-HH/CMR/4/32C/915.

412 DHC, NG-HH/CMR/4/32C/907.

413 DHC, NG-HH/CMR/4/32B/438.

414 DHC, NG-HH/CMR/4/13/1.

Lunacy Commissioners reported finding six lunatics at Blandford Forum, four at Poole, two at Wareham, eight at Weymouth and four at Wimborne Minster.[415] Probably, the lack of available places at Forston, and the increased costs associated with sending patients to Fisherton, meant that a review of inmates in these institutions was not a priority for the county.

Dorset's poor insane were fortunate, perhaps, that the public asylum opened relatively early which benefitted, at the same time, the all too poor communities who were subsidising their unaffordable care. This progress, as we know, signalled the end of private asylum care in the county and which may have contributed to the closure of Halstock asylum. Such a change also affected, in the late 1850s, the plight of the not so wealthy private patient. There is no evidence that any other new private asylums were emerging to make provision for these patients. John White tried but failed in 1843 at Stockland and Cranborne's William Symes had given up and moved to Southampton. The only other attempt to open a private asylum for eight ladies was made over 30 years later, in 1884, at Branksome Park on the coast near Poole; it failed due to local objections.[416]

The period from the mid-19th century must have caused difficulties for Dorset's non pauper insane. Some, as we know, followed William Symes out of the county and eventually to private provision in the Channel Islands. Others may have looked outside the county for accommodation where the private asylums, providing a much needed service, continued for much of the second half of the century.[417] The remainder, if manageable, may have found care in individual homes. It could be thought that the visiting officials at Herrison understood that provision for the non-pauper insane was lacking prompting their admittance to the public asylum in the early 1860s.

415   Rogers, *In the course of time*, p.18.
416   Brown, *A History of Dorset Hospitals*, p.171.
417   Parry-Jones, *Trade in Lunacy*, p.283.

CONCLUSION

T HE PRIVATE ASYLUMS placed in three Dorset villages were quite different from each other. The location of each shaped their characteristics and created individual histories. Each property lent itself for a specific style of its intended purpose.

The asylum at Cranborne was situated in the heart of the village whilst Halstock's asylum was just outside, with Stockland further away from the centre of the village. The Cranborne property had the luxury of house appeal, one of the grandest in the village and the ideal country house making it an attractive destination for those in need.

Cranborne appeared to be the most manageable asylum. William Symes, as proprietor, had chosen to take private patients only. This was not unusual, many madhouse proprietors did the same, creating a high class establishment where wealthier families could send their relatives.[418] The asylum building itself dictated this outcome or perhaps it was selected with this in mind. In any case unlike the other two asylums, it lacked the outbuildings in which to accommodate or confine pauper patients, neither was its position in the village conducive to such a plan. Having decided to take privately funded patients only, occasionally referred to as ladies and gentlemen by visiting magistrates, the resulting numbers were low in and patients were looked after by a relatively high ratio of staff. It seems likely that given the small number of patients due diligence would have been necessary to find those who would 'best fit' with the others whilst also needing to balance the books. Apart from one case, which was made known in the Quarter Sessions, Symes in this aspect seems to have been quite successful in creating a pleasant home.

The asylum and its daily activities, situated as it was in the centre of a fairly prosperous community, probably required constant daily consideration in respect of its neighbours. After initial objections it may always have been viewed with a mixture of suspicion and fear and never

---

418   Parry-Jones, *Trade in Lunacy*, p.56.

quite fully accepted. But no specific instances of tension between the asylum and the community were mentioned by the Visitors, beside a single instance in which the vicar banned a particularly disruptive patient from attending services. Not all the patients were 'easy', some were violent and needed to be restrained at times, but generally they appeared to have certain freedoms and were not imprisoned.

Symes' decision to leave Cranborne was probably born out of a combination of issues, he certainly would have liked to accommodate more patients, but the Quarter Sessions was always reluctant to grant a licence for him to do so. This may in turn have led to the financial difficulties which resulted in his court fees being overdue in 1842. Perhaps in the end, even with his farming sideline, the rewards were not as anticipated and moving out of the area with a business partner to a much larger and established asylum for both private and pauper patients offered, potentially, a more lucrative prospect.

Stockland, by contrast, confined more pauper patients than the other two private asylums. It was situated well away from the village which was probably taken into consideration when its licences were granted. The buildings seem to have been well suited with outbuildings and outside space. The high number of pauper patients was perhaps driven by the security that payment of fees by parish officials could be reasonably assured whereas the fees payable by the privately funded might be in arrears or defaulted. In this type of asylum expectations would be low, treatments barely considered, paupers locked up or restrained, lessening the need for many staff. However, they were almost certainly better that the standards found in many workhouses and unregulated lodgings provided in parishes for single patients.

William Spicer, Stockland asylum's proprietor, perhaps became overwhelmed by the relentless required paperwork and upkeep of the house. He seemed unable to manage the numbers of patients and provide the necessary distinction between paupers and private boarders which had been repeatedly requested by the Visitors. He could not have known, at the start of his establishment, that all things relating to running a private asylum would change quite so dramatically after only eight years. The new regulations and levels of inspection would have surely been challenging. It is hard to determine why any private patients were attracted to William Spicer's asylum and a strong presumption is that selection must have been based upon cost or location. Perhaps the promise of better things to come attracted the families of the three male private patients admitted between

1828 and 1832; one of whom was said to be a London barrister.

In the August of 1841 Spicer made a last ditch attempt to appease the court by pointing out that the management of the lunatics had been approved by a representative of the court of Chancery. But the wheels were already in motion and after just 21 years it was forcibly closed even though the need was evident. Had the asylum been able to continue it seems very likely that with the introduction of visits from the new Metropolitan Commissioners, courtesy of the Lunacy Act of 1842, any reprise under William Spicer would have been short lived. Perhaps the asylum would have fared better under its potential proprietor, John White, certainly he was endorsed in his quest by two Justices of the Peace, but ultimately he was apparently defeated by the level of renovation work required at the property.

Halstock attracted private patients alongside providing accommodation for paupers. The rented property was not ideal and maintaining such a large building caused many problems. It is a testament to the Mercer family, who appear to have been exemplary proprietors across several generations, that the asylum continued despite losses of key personnel. It seems likely that their general good standing in the village community contributed to its longevity.

The tension at Halstock between the capable asylum proprietors with inadequate facilities was highlighted in the report made in 1844 the Metropolitan Commissioners in Lunacy. It described Halstock's proprietor as one who was 'kindly disposed towards his patients' though criticised two of the occupied rooms as 'low, dirty and without any furniture except a wooden bedstead'.[419] Three years later in 1847 patients were asked whether they were comfortable or had any complaints. In response they expressed their gratitude for the kindness shown by Mr and Mrs Mercer. Ultimately the asylum, though long lasting, was not without its problems. Management was criticised on many occasions one of which was the inability, as at Stockland, to control the distinctions between the sexes and status of the patients and it too came close to losing its licence.

Across its 84 years about 293 people are known to have been admitted to Halstock asylum. There were 35 identifiable deaths, 26 people were moved to Forston, either immediately after discharge or some time later, and three were moved to asylums outside the county. Information relating to the remaining 229 patients was not recorded.

The asylums were small compared to others around the country. Halstock, the first to be licenced in 1774, grew it seems from a local surgeon

419   *Report of the Metropolitan Commissioners in Lunacy*, 1844) p.40.

caring for one or more privately funded patients at home. The same was probably the case for Stockland and Cranborne in the early 19th century. How the asylum 'trade' was learnt was not recorded, but local surgeons must have gained a range of experience both during their apprenticeships and as part of their daily business. Perhaps the asylum proprietors were familiar with the conditions and expectations associated with the workhouse and had some first hand experience of making provision under the poor laws as parish officials.

For Halstock virtually nothing is known of daily asylum life and treatments across its first 54 years, it was of no concern to the court of Quarter Sessions. Outside of the court changes to public attitudes were accelerated by the circumstances of George III and the focus placed on his insanity. Many treatments were tried and tested, the use of opiates to calm patients along with physical restraints and other forms of 'therapy' continued much as before. For the private asylum curing a patient as swiftly as possible remained the objective; success ensured a good reputation.

By the early 19th century knowledge of the new system known as the 'Moral' treatment, pioneered largely by the Tuke family at The Retreat in York, may well have reached the Mercer family and possibly even the visiting magistrates. Its approach was based on the belief that offering kindness and removing invasive medical methods, amongst other progressive concepts, would be effective.

Activities and occupations across the asylums were much the same, changing for the better over the years. The 'airing grounds', evident on the plans at Halstock and Stockland, were in use no doubt most days although comparisons have been made between these areas and of prescribed prison exercise in yards.[420] Gradually reports were made which noted patients out walking, gardening, sewing, reading, assisting in the kitchen and in the case of Stockland and Cranborne, spending time, sometimes in paid employment, at the various farms. Participation in divine service was an activity of sorts though it was more of a legal requirement. Whilst it is not documented it could be assumed that these activities were available to all classes, where able, of patients. Time away from the asylums which involved visits to family and friends was often recorded at Cranborne and, on occasion, at Halstock.

Aspects of personal care was rarely discussed. Reference to the provision of warm baths was made at Halstock only. House plans for Stockland shows bathing facilities though it seems unlikely these were

420   Brown, *A History of Dorset Hospitals*, p.162.

offered as a means of therapy; no such facility is expressed on the Cranborne plan. Cleanliness within the house was important along with ventilation which largely meant fresh air flow through the rooms and at Stockland the use of 'ventilators' was recommended. Further attempts to reduce the risk of illness involved the use of lime which the Visitors recommended at Halstock and Cranborne. That there were relatively few reports of infections resulting in deaths passing through all three houses was remarkable.

Speed of intervention and some sort of curative treatment were both recognised as essential if there was any hope to cure insanity. This became the subject of many a debate in parliament committees as the realisation that people locked away had no chance of recovery and only became worse as time passed. Private patients living in small home-like establishments like Cranborne with attention to their everyday needs fared better and some were discharged 'cured', but were frequently re-admitted with a few patients remaining in some sort of care all their lives. In all three asylums the sample sizes are too small and the records too limited to provide any analysis of their relative success in facilitating cures.

The term incurable was often used to signify failure of being cured within 12 months. Generally, this meant that pauper patients said to be incurable after a year, were removed from private or public asylums into cheap custody elsewhere.[421] This was true for Bethlem and St Luke's where long standing cases were not admitted and kept none for more than a year.[422] There is little evidence of this at Halstock or Stockland and, although records are patchy, many remained for years.

It is likely that those who were classed as insane and curable, enjoyed better conditions and treatment than who were pronounced 'idiots' from birth. Those amongst the parish poor born with abnormalities were not usually worth the expense of private asylum care and may have been also rejected by the asylum proprietors. Their fate was confinement in the workhouse or at home receiving parish relief. Only a handful of people were described as such in the Dorset asylums. No mention has been found concerning individuals with physical disabilities.

There were few institutions country wide specialising in the care of idiots or minors within the private madhouse system during the first half of the 19th century.[423] Gradually the situation changed bringing a small school for idiotic children in Bath in 1846. Towards the end of the 19th century

---

421 Parry-Jones, *The Trade in Lunacy*, pp.198-9.

422 Ibid., p.198.

423 Ibid., p.70.

four licenced houses across the country had been established focussing entirely in the care of idiots.[424]

Inconsistent record keeping means that it is only possible to determine the length of time spent in the asylum for a small number of patients. The time spent in confinement varied widely. For some it could be a matter of months, for others a number of years. One of the longest periods spent at Halstock was that of Captain John Spong, gentleman, from Wimborne Minster. He remained in the asylum from 1779, aged 50 to his burial in 1806 at Halstock 27 years later.[425]

The involvement of family and friends in the treatment and care of private patients is particularly difficult to establish. Edward Phelips, a member of the Phelips family of Montacute,[426] was an asylum patient identified and buried without fanfare at Halstock. Born in 1789, the third child of seven, to the Revd William Phelips and Anna Aletheia Elizabetha, he had been committed to Halstock in 1825 by his brothers, Robert and Richard, both members of the clergy. He spent 23 years at the asylum before his death from influenza in 1848.[427] Edward's father made no mention of him in his will, but in a codicil to his mother's will, dated March, 1814, she bequeathed 'for his sole benefit all my wines spirits with the bottles'. In a later codicil dated May 1814 this was revoked. It was presumably thought to be an ill advised gift to her 25 year old son, and it appears that she also revoked her bequest of a bed, bedstead and furniture. Instead she left him her horses and carriage for 'his sole use'.[428] As in so many cases there is not enough detail to understand the nature of Edward's condition and care.

Was it worth the effort? Parish officials in 1800 paid between 9s. and 12s. per week for the keep of pauper lunatics; in 1816 the Mercer family at Halstock charged 12s. for basic weekly board. Fees for private patients varied according to individual requirements and 'amenities' on offer. Surprisingly perhaps, only two private patient cases at Halstock were officially recorded for non or late payment of fees.

Regular asylum outgoing financial costs were the annual licence fees of £10 or £15, food provision and a level of furniture and bedding. Clothing for the poor was normally supplied by their 'friends', the parish officials, which were sometimes found woefully inadequate by the Visitors. Private

424   Ibid., p.72.
425   DHC, PE-HAL/RE/1/2.
426   *Burke's Landed Gentry*, v. II (1879), pp.1265-6.
427   DHC, PE-HAL/RE/4/1.
428   TNA, PROB 11/1590/29. Piece 1590.

patients may have had disposable money of their own and some may have participated in paid work. To some extent they had the financial capacity to meet any personal requirements which were not provided as part of their package of care. This benefit was probably not available, officially at least, to the pauper patients.

Staff were rarely mentioned either in terms of qualities required, subsequent training, or wages. The census returns of 1841 and 1851 show that those employed of resident staff and servants were mostly young, inexperienced, relatively cheap labour. Almost all of the staff were from the locality of their respective asylums. In 1841 Stockland showed three staff, the keeper (manager) aged 24 and two domestic servants under 20 years of age with 21 patients under their care. The same census reveals Halstock with four servants, three in their twenties, looking after eight patients. Ten years later the asylum employed two staff both aged 19 for four patients. In contrast the 1841 census for Cranborne boasted four assistants, all aged 20, for six private patients. The proprietors presumably provided additional assistance and were described in each setting in 1841, as resident medical attendant (Halstock) resident surgeon (Cranborne) and governor (Stockland). In all asylums, and particularly in those like Stockland whose patient base was largely made up of paupers, staff expenses were kept to a minimum. There was fine line between keeping parish maintenance payments as low as possible and profit.[429]

It was not until the early to mid-19th century that the qualities and training of staff began to be considered. Gradually the importance of good and trustworthy staff was understood to be a major factor towards improvements within the private asylum system and in 1843 formal nurse training in psychiatry took place for the first time at Surrey County Asylum.[430] The success and reputation of private asylums relied on recruiting good male attendants and it was realised that difficulties retaining them was broadly down to inadequate pay. No details of these issues survive for the Dorset asylums, any improvements and changes in this respect were most likely taking place at some distance away. For employees in Dorset any 'training' occurred in the workplace and recruitment was made from those who were prepared to do what was required.

While wages in the private asylums went unrecorded, they are available for the newly opened Forston county asylum. At the outset, in 1832, for the period June to September, male attendants received £6 5s. and female attendants £3 15s. The cook and laundry attendant each received

429   Parry-Jones, *The Trade in Lunacy*, pp.186-7.
430   Ibid., p.186.

£3.[431] It could be presumed that similar wage rates may have been paid at Cranborne asylum with rather less, perhaps, at the other asylums.

Since all three private asylums were usually managed by surgeons it was only necessary to buy in medical assistance at Halstock when Alice and Harriett Mercer were the designated proprietors. At other times there was a resident surgeon available on site which provided a both a financial saving and benefit to patients.

As a business Halstock seems to have been the most successful. It survived the shocks of the deaths of two proprietors, one of whom was in recovery from a devastating fire. The women who managed the asylum dealt with these adverse conditions and at no time was their financial stability called into question by the visiting authorities.

Visits by court officials, physicians, accommodation and travel expenses were covered by the court as was the subsequent reporting costs undertaken by the court clerk.

Law changes and impact

The impact of increased inspections in 1828 from one to four a year can only be imagined. For Halstock, particularly after 53 years and Stockland, after a mere eight years, the prospect of any inspections must have been considered a nuisance, perhaps a worry, and probably unwelcome. For the pauper patients it may have afforded some opportunity to have concerns addressed. It is clear that both Visitors and Commissioners spoke to the patients and sometimes took action upon what they heard.

Advance notification of the new regulations was made known ahead of the Visitors' first inspection, but it appears that the Mercer's at Halstock were unprepared. Presumably the same notification was issued to Stockland. As time went by it seems that the proprietors of Halstock acted upon the recommendations made by the Visitors, whereas at Stockland there was less inclination to do so.

Visitors constantly criticised all three asylum keepers for their inability to provide the required paperwork, excuses were often made, some quite imploring in tone. For Stockland and Cranborne failure to comply with the required record keeping might be seen as a major contributing factor to their eventual closures. It is not known why maintaining registers proved to be such a problem, however the Dorset asylums were not alone, it was a widespread offence across the country.[432]

431   DHC, D-1430/1/1.
432   Parry-Jones, *The Trade in Lunacy*, p.263.

In part the 1828 Lunacy Act had been introduced to prevent the improper confinement of sane people who had been deprived of their liberty. The reputation held by private asylums, derived from the fear of improper confinement, was for corrupt motives of mercenary proprietors and corrupt medical men.[433] But, this does not appear to have been a problem that afflicted any of the Dorset asylums. Only one patient, at Halstock, was deemed to have been incarcerated without due cause and his wife pleaded with the authorities to maintain his confinement. Otherwise, where the Visitors or physicians requested a patient's release following a 'cure', a trial period was often suggested.

In other areas suggestions made by the Visitors were acted upon; demonstrating that they had some power to instigate change. Spicer, the proprietor at Stockland, responded to the request for better ventilation in 1829. Symes, keeper at Cranborne, placed iron bars in some bedrooms in 1831, although initially he had expressed some reluctance to do so, and the Mercers at Halstock, provided a bath for patients within weeks of its suggestion in 1828.

Each asylum was visited by the same group of local Justices of the Peace, no individual is known to have officially attended or reported on more than one establishment. From 1842 and the passing of the Lunacy Act, the Halstock and Cranborne asylums were inspected by the Commissioners in Lunacy. These were the same individuals for both asylums and they brought with them experience of visiting institutions in other counties. This provided the consistency which the Act's creators had hoped to achieve. Stockland and importantly its patients, did not benefit from this level of attention as the asylum by this time had closed.

The Commissioners in Lunacy introduced some degree of uniformity into the management of patients and into the conditions in provincial houses.[434] They demonstrated the advantages of regular visits and inspection from a body of men who were experienced, and who were beyond suspicion of local partiality. Prior to this the visiting magistrates and medical Visitors were probably ignorant of the provisions and purposes of the lunacy laws and their inexperience rendered them ill suited to give opinions on care and management. It was said, as indicated in Oxfordshire records, that Visitors often failed in their statutory duties and also in the adequacy of their inspections. Nevertheless, their contribution cannot be disregarded.

433   Ibid., p.290.
434   Ibid., p.290-1.

Reports differed, sometimes quite considerably, between the local Visiting Justices and the Commissioners. The Justices who visited the private asylums in their capacity as appointed representatives of the court no doubt had many other demands on their time and, of these, only a small minority had some knowledge of the subject. The Visitors received very little in terms of guidance on the subject, particularly in respect of the Madhouse Act of 1828, apart from recommendations to observe the provision of religious activities in the house.[435] The Commissioners constituted a different inspection altogether, many had been appointed because of their knowledge and their collective mission for change. This greater knowledge and enhanced remit was evident in their reports.

Levels of success for curing the insane are not easy to determine. The Quarter Session records the outcomes of many patients, but some remain unknown and some were not recorded at all. All expressions used for patients leaving the asylum are self explanatory except perhaps for the term 'relieved' which is understood to mean being relieved of their burden or immediate distress. This 'relief' was often short lived with sufferers returning to the same asylum or found later admitted to Forston.

Reasons for insanity were seldom stated and those mentioned were usually 'epilepsy' and 'idiot'. The nature and some causes of mental illness can be discovered, though much later, through the order (admission) papers for those committed to Forston. In 1849 these included 'excitement', 'poverty', 'domestic unhappiness', 'disappointed views', 'childbirth', 'travelling by rail', 'grief' and 'injury to the head'.[436] This last cause was sometimes noted in cases admitted from the private asylums usually in terms of 'blow to the head'.

Other order papers for patients admitted to Forston who had previously been at Stockland show causes to be sudden fright, anxiety, (usually in respect of concerns about their children), dementia, state of mortal derangement, son going to Crimea, epilepsy, hereditary, drinking, and hereditary syphilis. For those who had formerly been at Halstock they were a master's suicide, typhus and nervous excitement, this last probably better described today as being anxious or in a state of panic. One of the strangest causes was given in respect of Mary Spear who had 'caught a cold in the head'.

Some were noted to be a 'dangerous lunatic', many were 'violent' and some were said to be suffering from 'no known cause'. Only three people

435   Ibid., p.298.
436   Rogers, *In the Course of Time*, p.17.

identified as 'idiots' or 'of weak intellect' appear to have been confined in the asylums.

The County Lunatic Asylum at Forston opened in 1832, earlier than most, and two decades before those in adjacent counties. Such was the response it filled up quickly. This was an inevitable outcome given that reports made by the committee were published in the press which pointed out that a lower rate was charged compared to the rate at private asylums. In addition, they were keen to press home the fact that there was no extra fee for medicine and clothing, a cost which was normally placed on pauper patients and their parishes in private establishments. No doubt, as a result just three years later, parish overseers were notified in the press that the asylum was nearly full and were directed by the visiting magistrates to check if places were available a week in advance.[437]

When the private asylums folded they were not replaced. This was probably because once the county system had been established nobody was prepared to make the necessary speculative investment for an institution that would only house private patients. This left a significant lack of provision which was for the most part filled by the Wiltshire private asylums at Fisherton and Laverstock until the construction of the new buildings at Herrison.

Much has been written of the adverse conditions prevailing in the private asylums.[438] Yet such condemnation needs to be considered alongside attitudes of the day towards insanity, strange behaviours and differences or social conditions in general. By today's standards treatments seem disproportionately harsh and brutal. Yet the belief that insanity had to be overcome by restraint and physical treatments was, by the late eighteenth and early nineteenth centuries, slowly evolving giving way to an era of different and kinder forms of treatment.

Over 400 patients passed through the Dorset private asylums over a collective 83 years. Some stayed whether willingly or otherwise for years, some just a few months. Maybe for some of the proprietors, it was a 'trade in lunacy' or maybe it was personal vocation with a philanthropic element. In any event it cannot have been an easy way to earn a living. Halstock kept going when the proprietors could have walked away, at Stockland the proprietor might have continued for longer had he not burnt his bridges with the court, and Cranborne, with so few patients, never seems to have had sufficient income to become securely established.

---

437 *Dorset County Chronicle,* 9 April 1835.

438 Parry-Jones, *Trade in Lunacy,* pp. 289-90.

For Dorset and its neighbouring counties Somerset, Wiltshire and Devon, living conditions for the majority of the population at this time was grim. Families suffered daily, a situation made immeasurably worse by behaviours displayed, often violent, by their loved ones. Therefore, it could be said that during their lifetime, and despite many difficulties, the Dorset private asylums provided a considerable public service. They were the only type of institution which offered some kind of comprehensive care of those afflicted with insanity in all its forms.[439] When choices were limited, and usually dire, some comfort may have been drawn from their existence.

In some cases no cause could be ascertained for the mental disorder. This fact increases the mystery with which Insanity is yet enveloped. It may indeed be affirmed, that men walk in shadow and darkness, whilst an inexorable abyss lies yawning under their feet - an abyss, which spares neither rich nor poor, neither learned nor unlearned, neither unenlighted nor wise.[440]

Dr G Button,
Forston asylum resident physician and superintendent.

439　Ibid., p.283.
440　DHC, NH-HH/CMR/2/1/2.

Case Studies

1. Amelia Lindquist, private patient and
bereaved mother.

O NE CASE STANDS out among the Halstock patients. It is that of Amelia Lindquist, who was born in Calcutta in 1813 and died at Bethnal asylum (Bedlam) in 1887.

Amelia Lindquist was a frequent private patient at Halstock. Her story began in Calcutta when the 16 year old Amelia Cohen married William Lindquist, a marine in the East India Bengal service, in July 1829.[441] William was described as being 'of age', Amelia 'under age'. Two years later the first of three children, Amelia, was born in Calcutta, who subsequently died in 1831 aged one, Diana was born in 1834 and Christiana in 1836. It is possible that another child was born in Calcutta around 1832/33 as there is a burial record for a William Henry Lindquist in the Wyke Regis parish registers dated 28 March 1836, he was 3½ years old.[442] In 1836 the family had relocated to Wyke Regis, Dorset where another child bearing the same name, William Henry, was born 17 March 1838.[443]

Amelia first entered the Halstock asylum when it was managed by Harriet Mercer. It is not clear when she was admitted, although it seems likely it was after the birth of her son in 1838. Having been released in March 1839, she was readmitted shortly afterwards and released again in June 1839. Her third admission was in November 1839 after which she was removed to a private house under care of Miss Mercer (probably Betsy, Harriet Mercer's aunt) within the village. The Quarter Session registers do not show when she was discharged from Halstock, presumably pregnant at the time, as in

---

441　Presidency of Bengal, parish register transcripts, 1713 - 1848 (N-1-24, British India Office Marriages, Lindquist and Cohen, 7 February 1829).

442　DHC, PE-WYK/RE/4/2.

443　DHC, PE-WYK/RE/2/4.

April 1840 a baptism for their son Horatio took place at Wyke Regis.[444] The census in the following year shows Amelia in Wyke Regis with husband William and two sons William and Horatio.[445] Her husband William was a man of some standing and was described as a 'gentleman' when he met the property qualification to be included on the Quarter Sessions list of prospective jurors for Radipole parish in 1840.[446]

The census also shows their daughters Diana and Christiana at a boarding school in Wyke Regis in 1841 when they were seven and six years old respectively.[447] It was their schoolmistress, Mary Twigg, who signed a printed admission notice to place their mother Amelia, then aged 33, once again in Halstock in August 1846. The admission notice gave her previous places of confinement as Halstock, Earls Court and Brompton. John Justinian Mercer's report added that she was 'in a tranquil state of mind but subject to great incoherence in her language' and not in good bodily health. Her admission was recorded in the new countrywide register for lunacy patients, the Lunacy Admission Register, maintained by the Lunacy Commission.[448] She remained at Halstock for over two years and was discharged in January of 1849 'not improved'.

During this time she caused a scandal by giving birth to a child at Halstock asylum. The father was unknown. At the time the Visitors said 'Mrs Mercer cannot account for such an occurrence having taken place in the asylum, and says she has no suspicion or clue as to the father of this child'. She stated that the patient had escaped over some gates on two occasions and was absent some time. The child, Amelia, was baptised in Halstock on 9 November 1848, when her mother was described in the parish register as 'a patient in Halstock lunatic asylum'.[449]

The incident was exceptional and reported in the press in January 1849:[450]

> Extraordinary Case - On Tuesday, the Dorsetshire sessions, Mr Sheridan, MP called the attention of the Court to the most unfortunate circumstance

444   Ibid.
445   *Census* 1841.
446   DHC, Q/S/J/5/1840/107.
447   *Census*, 1841.
448   TNA, MH/94/7.
449   DHC, PE-HAL/RE/2/1.
450   *Taunton Courier and Western Advertiser*, 17 January 1849.

that had recently occurred at the Halstock Private Lunatic Asylum a circumstance which he mentioned as one of the visitors of that asylum, and on which the metropolitan Commissioners had made a special report. Mr Sheridan then proceeded to read from the report the Commissioners Dr Prichard and Mr Proctor, the details of the circumstance alluded to A Mrs ---- was two years ago admitted into this asylum as a patient, her husband being abroad. In the course of the winter she managed to escape from the asylum but she was brought back by a female servant before she had been away an hour. No suspicion of any impropriety had been entertained, nor was any person observed near her, yet the unfortunate lady proved pregnant, and was delivered in the asylum of child of whose parentage not the most distant idea could be formed. Mr Sheridan after reading the report said the justices had the power if they thought fit of recommending to the Lord Chancellor that the licence should be revoked, but seeing how well the house had been conducted and much it had been improved of late, he certainly would not advise that such a step should be taken.

After some discussion the Clerk of the Peace was directed to make a special minute of the matter.

Additional information was recorded in the Sherborne Mercury in January 1849. It stated that Mr Mercer, who had died before the child was born, had known of the situation but had failed to report it as he should have done. The Commissioners acquitted Mrs Mercer of all blame, but criticism was made that there appeared to be no 'proper means of separating the males from the females'. The report continued that Mr Sheridan had been at the asylum when the patient made a similar escape and when she was returned she 'again got out of the room and concealed herself in the apartments of the males.' Mrs Mercer was to be called upon to make an efficient separation.

Amelia Lindquist was discharged at the end of January 1849, although her condition was said to be 'not improved'.[451] The discharge took place on the 'wish of Mrs Mercer who states that she was too difficult a patient to manage' and no record was made of her immediate movements thereafter. By 1852 she was again in London and noted to be a lunatic when her daughter was baptised in October for a second time at Chilthorne Domer, Somerset.[452] William Linquest (sic) gentleman, and Amelia were recorded as the parents although it remained uncertain that he was the child's true father and at the time of the baptism William was away at sea. The census

451   TNA, MH/94/7.
452   SHC, D/P/chi.dom/2/1/6.

Mr. Sheridan, as one of the Visiting Justices, presented a report of the commissioners of Lunacy, respecting a painful circumstance which occurred at the Halstock asylum. One of the unfortunate inmates, a lady, having made her escape from the house, was pursued and, after a time was discovered, and brought back. Subsequently it was discovered that she was pregnant; but the circumstance was not reported to the Visiting Justices until the child was born. The commissioners in lunacy as soon as they heard of the matter, caused an investigation to be made, and the report was now presented to the court for consideration. It appeared that Mr. Mercer, who died before the child was born, was aware of the circumstance, but neglected to report it as he ought to have done. The child was born on the 15th of October last. Mr. Sheridan observed that the commissioners acquitted Mrs. Mercer of all blame; but there did not appear to be at the asylum, proper means of separating the males from the females. While he (Mr. Sheridan) was there the patient made her escape in a similar manner, and on being brought back, she again got out of the room and concealed herself in the apartments of the males.

The Rev. J. A. Templar, was of opinion that Mrs. Mercer should be called upon to make an efficient separation between male and female patients.

The court directed that the Clerk of the Peace should make a special minute of the case, and write to Mrs. Mercer about it.

The incident at Halstock asylum concerning Amelia Lindquist was reported in the Sherborne Mercury in January 1849. Details of the affair were made public in a report of the Commissioners of Lunacy and read to the Quarter Session court by Richard B. Sheridan who was one of the Visiting Justices. The essence of the criticism related to the fact that the asylum building was not conducive to keep male and female patients apart though no blame was placed on Harriet Mercer.

conducted the previous year revealed the child Amelia Lindquist was living with the Bengefield family in Chilthorne Domer, a few miles north of Halstock. In years to come the younger Amelia benefitted from a bequest made in Harriet Mercer's will of £5 which was accompanied by the words 'and her receipt alone shall be sufficient discharge and independent of any husband with whom she may intermarry'.[453]

453   DHC, NG-PB/1/8/26.

The exact whereabouts of Amelia's incarceration after 1849 is unknown. The Lunacy Patients Admission Registers recorded her 18 years later in August 1867 when she was admitted to Bethnal House, in a private capacity, where she remained until her death some 20 years later in October 1887 at the age of 74.[454]

2. JOSEPH WHITROW, PAUPER PATIENT AND CRIMINAL LUNATIC

JOSEPH WHITROW, FROM the small coastal parish of Kimmeridge, appeared at the court of Quarter Sessions in February 1814. The register recorded his age as 32, single and a labourer, he had been committed by J. Calcraft esquire accused of 'threatening to kill William Clavell esquire and Sophia his wife' the outcome of which was to secure sureties himself of £40 for one year and two sureties in £20 each. He was discharged but detained again on another charge of the same complainant.[455] An earlier record was made in the Quarter Session Order book with an entry dated 1813 which reported that sureties had been filed for Joseph Whiterow to keep the peace and be of good behaviour towards 'all his Majesty's liege subjects' and especially towards the said William Clavell for one year and then to be discharged. [456]

In April 1815 he was back in court this time for a breach of peace. The prison register described him as 'orderly' and he was asked again to find sureties for two calendar months. He was discharged in September 1815 and taken off to Halstock by Mr Edward Parmiter of Kimmeridge Farm.[457]

The Quarter Session Order book also recorded Joseph Whitrow within the Calendar of Prisoners in September 1815. Articles of the peace having been exhibited received and filed against him on the oath of William Clavell esquire ordered that he be imprisoned in the house of correction of the county for the space of two 'calenday months' and then to be discharged.[458]

The Kimmeridge parish relief account book confirms Joseph's confinement at the asylum where the overseers paid his board in 1816 for

454   TNA, MH 94/7.
455   DHC, NG-PR/1/D/2/1.
456   DHC, Q/S/M/1/14, f. 88.
457   DHC, NG-PR/1/D/2/1.
458   DHC, Q/S/M/1/14, f. 154.

30 weeks to 'Mr Mercer of Halstock' at 7s. per week, the sum of £10 10s.[459]
By March 1818 this fee had reduced to 5s. per week for a year's board at the
asylum, a total of £13. The same applied in the following year but there was
no entry made in 1820. Joseph Whitrow had consistently been named on
the asylum register from September 1815, annually, but by August 1819 his
name had been removed. The 5s. fee paid by Kimmeridge parish to Halstock,
is clearly a much reduced rate compared to the 12s. paid in respect of Mary
Curtis of Puddletown during the same year of 1816. Perhaps the shortfall
was made up by the court or perhaps the fee reflected the level of care he
received at Halstock.

It appears that Joseph Whitrow was returned to Kimmeridge as his
name reappears in Kimmeridge poor accounts in March 1820, here the
parish paid 'Ambrose Furber for Joseph Whitrow' £10, presumably for
looking after him over 50 weeks.[460] This arrangement continued, in 1822 Mr
Furber received £6 7s. 6d. for half of 51 weeks at 5s. per week.

The Kimmeridge overseers of the poor made two further payments for
the care of Joseph Whitrow in 1830 to Susan Silby, one for looking after him
during the winter, 7s. and another of 10s. for waiting on him during his illness.
The same year saw payments for Joseph Whitrow's coffin and furniture, £1;
for digging the grave and tolling the bell 6s. His burial was recorded in the
Church Knowle parish register in September 1830; he was 53.[461]

3. MARY CURTIS, PAUPER PATIENT, GRIEVING WIDOW

A LETTER FROM the asylum proprietor John Mercer to Thomas Banger, an
overseer in Puddletown, in the September of 1816 gives some insight into
how the admission process for paupers might operate.[462] Mercer wrote that
the asylum had a vacancy and a female pauper could be received at any time.
She was expected to bring her own clothing (provided by the parish) and he
specified that she should bring five shifts 'and other things in proportion'. His
letter concludes with financial considerations and the costs which the parish
overseers would be expected to meet: for entrance £1 1s. 0d., board for each
week 12s., and medicine £5 5s. 0d. The charge for medicine was presumably
an estimate and might vary according to future treatment as it was to be paid

---

459   DHC, D-689/1.
460   Ibid..
461   DHC, PE-CKL/RE/4/2.
462   DHC, PE-PUD/OV/7/5.

John Mercer's letter to Thomas Banger, overseer at Puddletown, advising of a vacancy at Halstock asylum and detailing the costs involved, 1816. DHC, PE-PUD/OV/7/5.

when the patient left the asylum. No name was given in the letter but a Mary Curtis, from Puddletown appeared on the Halstock register in April 1817. Account records of the Puddletown overseers confirm the parish paid for her to be confined at Halstock in September 1816 at a cost of 12s. per week. Another document shows a bill paid to E. Stickland for 'the time widow Curtis remained in his house' - 10s. for ten weeks.[463]

463   DHC, PE-PUD/OV/1/54/9.

Sir,

I did not receive your favour this last evening respecting a female pauper, the terms for that class I have stated as underneath -

There being a vacancy, one can receive her any day that should prove most convenient for you to remove her. It is necessary for her to be provided with a proper quantity of Living viz: 5 Shifts and other things in proportion.

> I remain Sir
>
> > Your most obediant........?
> >
> > > John Mercer

Portland Cottage

11 September 1816

Entrance - £1 1[s.] o[d.] p[ai]d by T Banger, entered on account

Board for week - 12[s.]

Medicine - 5[s.] 5[d.]

The medicine but one charge to be paid at the time the patient leaves the asylum

Another entry shows a bill for the board at the asylum for the widow Curtis from 19 September 1816 to April 1817 which amounted to £16 16s. Added to this were the cost of shoes and clothing making a total of £18 2s 6d. [464] The following bill accounted for the year from April 1817 to March 1818, the basic weekly cost remained at 12s. added to which were costs for clothes, shoes and mending making a total of £35 18s. 9½d. [465] John Mercer accompanied the bill dated March 1818 with a note,

> Respecting her present state I have to observe that her bodily health is perfectly restored, in regard to her state of mind I cannot pronounce her perfect. She being at times very irritable, was (you) to remove her I fear you would find her at times a troublesome person.

Less than two months later John Mercer was dead, a tragic event which appeared to have consequences for Mary as can be seen by the following letter written by Betsy Mercer to the parish officials in July 1818:

464   DHC, PE-PUD/OV/1/54/1.
465   DHC, PE-PUD/OV/1/56/4.

'In consequence of the decease of my brother in law (John Mercer) I have taken the liberty of forwarding the amount of Mrs Curtis's board and up to the period of my late friends death, in which I have included the charge specified for medicines on her arrival here to match (same) finally to close the books of the establishment with the death of the late Mr Mercer. May I therefore request an early remittance of the amount.' [466]

The bill was £57 7s. 0d., including the £5 5s. 'to match' covering the period April 1817 to September 1818.

From this it appears that Alice, John Mercer's widow, with a child just a year old, had decided at the time to close the asylum. Mary Curtis disappeared from the Halstock records without further comment but she can be found again amongst paupers named in the Puddletown overseers in 1819 showing payments of £1 4s. being paid to her on a monthly basis. [467] Further unspecified expenses of 15s. were paid to Halstock for widow Curtis in the same year along with 'house rents Mr Alner, for widow Curtis 15s. for half a year'.

It seems she was returned to her home parish where she stayed for a number of years before being admitted to the recently opened county asylum at Forston in 1834, aged 62. [468] Her order paper stated that she was from Puddletown, a widow with two children and the cause of her insanity was said to be 'nervous excitement'. Eight years later, in March 1842, a Forston case register and order (admittance) paper show Mary Curtis, a dressmaker now aged 70, admitted once again. [469] By December that year she had been released though returned less than three years later in May 1845. [470] More details of her condition were given this time. Her character was described as temperate, sanguine, kind and of good intellect, she could read and write; her accompanying bodily disorder was described as 'derangement of digestive functions'. She had suffered with ill health and poverty and grief all of which contributed to the cause of her mental disorder; she was buried in Puddletown, aged 73. [471]

---

466   DHC, PE-PUD/OV/1/56/12.

467   DHC, PE-PUD/OV/1/6.

468   DHC, NG-HH/CMR/4/32A/106.

469   DHC, NG-HH/CMR/4/32A/106 (1834), NG-HH/CMR/4/32B/346 (1842) and NG-HH/CMR/4/13/1.

470   DHC, NG-HH/CMR/4/13/1.

471   DHC, PE-PUD/RE/4/2.

APPENDIX 1.

NUMBERS OF PATIENTS attending private asylums where numbers are available for complete calendar years, 1775-1855.[472]

Figure 1. Halstock, male patients, 1775-1855, five year average plotted on the central year.

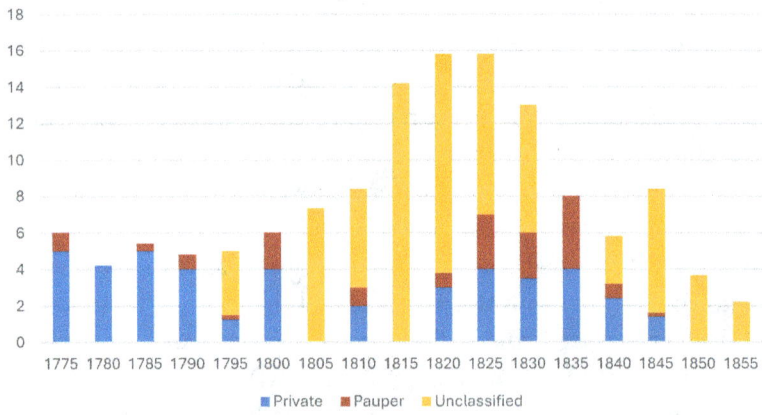

Figure 2. Halstock, female patients, 1775-1855, five year average plotted on the central year.

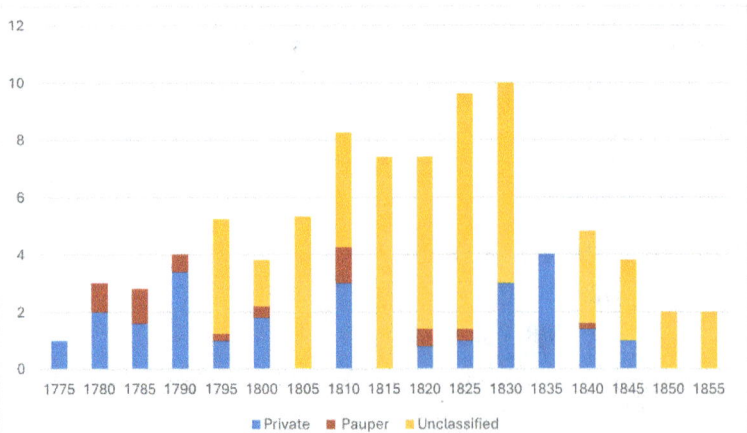

472   DHC, Q/A/L/Private/1.

Figure 3. Stockland, male patients, 1820-1841.[473]

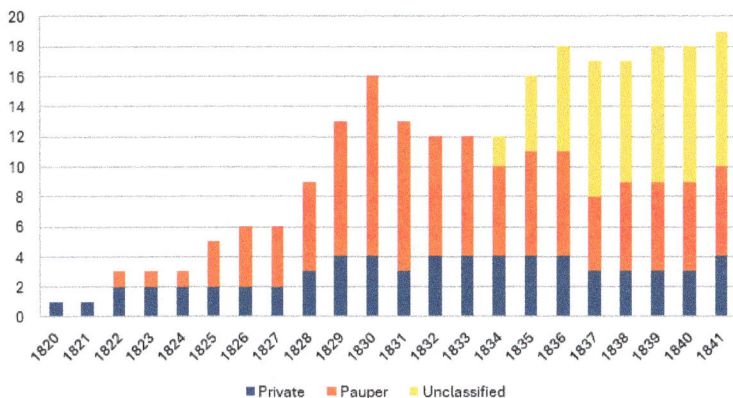

Private   Pauper   Unclassified

Figure 4. Stockland, female patients, 1820-1841.

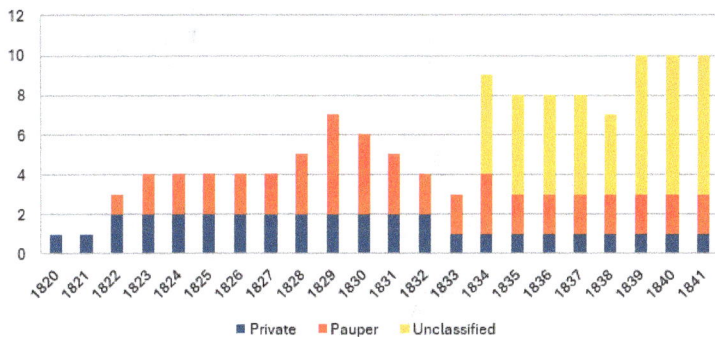

Private   Pauper   Unclassified

Figure 5. Cranborne, private male and female patients, 1827-1848. [474]

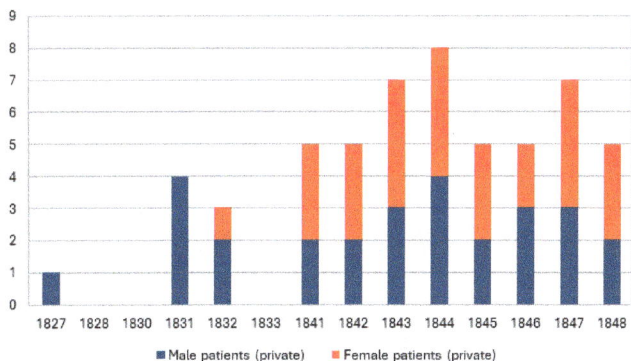

Male patients (private)   Female patients (private)

473   DHC, Q/A/L/Private/1.

474   DHC, Q/A/L/Private/1.

Forston patients, 1832-1868, for those years where year end totals are available, with numbers of admissions by sex where available (all pauper except in 1865)[475]

Date	Male admissions in year	Female admissions in year	Male total patients at end of year	Female total patients at end of year	Total patients remaining at end of year	Additional patients housed at Fisherton, Wilts.
1832					35	
1834			33	36	69	
1835			38	41	79	
1837	10	16			100	
1839	11	17			103	
1840	9	16			108	
1841					98	
1842			52	61	113	
1843					107	
1844			51	67	118	
1849			65	87	153	
1850			69	92	161	
1851			72	93	165	
1852	19	17			155	
1853			72	86	158	
1856			69	88	157	
1858			70	88	158	
1859			76	93	169	70
1863			111	101	212	69
1864			129	147	276	
1865			139	149	288*	
1866			147	160	307	

* Total includes one non pauper patient from outside Dorset and eight from Dorset.

APPENDIX 2.

The list of patients is likely to be incomplete as full registers were not always maintained. Misspellings and mishearing names and places appear to be common. Some people may be listed more than once with a different home parish. Dates show the year of admittance or when first recorded in the registers and files retained by the Quarter Sessions.

Cranborne patients		
Almond, James	Jersey, Channel Islands	1844
Beale, Charles	Cambridge	1830
Blandford, Charlotte	Fifield Bavant, Wiltshire	1836
Blandford, Mary Ann	Fifield Bavant, Wiltshire	1836
Corbin, William	Shapwick	1833
Dale, Frederick Duodecimus	Brighton	1827
Ferris, John	Weymouth	1834
Foss, James	Blandford	1830
Gilbert, Fanny	Moor Crichel	1844
Green, Elizabeth	Blandford	1846
Hallett, George	unknown	1847
Henning, Thomas Parr	Alton Pancras	1847
Lanning, Jane	Corfe Mullen	1842
Lloyd, Edward	Jersey, Channel Islands	1847
Nation, Elizabeth	Blandford	1847
Oakley, Jane	Blandford	1840
Pond, James Fowler	Blandford	1843
Simmonds, Susannah	Wimborne	1831
Smith, Gould	Blandford	1830

Halstock patients		
Abbott, Edward	Bradford Abbas	1813
Adams, Ann	Burnham (Burnham-on-Sea), Somerset	1791
Andress, Ann	Bridport	1820
Andrews, Miss Betty	South Brent, Somerset	1775
Andrews, Cain	South Brent, Somerset	1775
Appleby, George	West Lydford, Somerset	1830
Baddon, John	Lothers (Loders)	1783
Bagwell, Nicholas	Beer, Devon	1795
Banger, Edmund	Lillington	1840
Barnes, Jane	Meere, (Meare) Somerset	1802
Barnes, Jane	Meere, (Mere) Wiltshire	1811
Barnes, Jane	Chideock	1814
Barnes, Samuel	Chideock	1815
Barrett, Thomas	Frampton	1815
Bartlett, Ann	Sandford, Somerset	1794
Bartlett, Edmund	Portesham	1823
Bartlett, Henry	Winterborne Abbas or Langton Herring	1832
Bartlett, Martha	Langton	1814
Bartlett, Thomas	Yeovil Marsh, Somerset	1775
Beaton, Charles	Yeovil, Somerset	1809
Beer, Isaac	Isle Abbotts, Somerset	1783
Belbin, Samuel	Yetminster	1828
Bennett, Rebecca	Upwey	1805
Berkeley, Jane	Yeovil, Somerset	1838
Best, Mary	Tyneham	1827
Bingham, George	Over Compton	1797
Bishop, Ann	Cattistock	1791
Bishop, Jane	Axminster, Devon	1812
Bishop, Mr	Ilminster, Somerset	1802
Bishop, Samuel	Axminster, Devon	1812
Bishop, William	Lothers (Loders)	1814
Blandy, John	Bradford Peverell	1811/1816
Blandy, Mr	Linkenholt, Hampshire	1824
Bonney, John	West Lulworth	1828

Bortland, Eleanor	Wareham	1816
Boswell, George Junior	Puddletown	1790
Brand, John	Topsham, Devon	1794
Brown, Elizabeth	Milborne Port, Somerset	1775
Browne, Mrs, Wife of John Browne	Exeter, Devon	1775
Budden, John	Lothers (Loders)	1783
Budge, Martha	Crewkerne, Somerset	1835
Budgell, John	unknown	1834
Burgess/Burges/Burge, Sarah	Castle Cary, Somerset	1775
Butter/Butler, Benjamin	Woodbury, Devon	1800
Cary, Mary	Downton, Somerset	1780
Cattle, Jane	Affpuddle	1797
Charles, Mrs	Osmington	1810
Childs, Robert	Whitcombe	1832
Chutter/Chubb/Cluth, Edward	Evershot, Dorset	1813
Clark, Sarah	Hazelbury, Somerset	1823
Clarke, Revd William	Perris Hill, Somerset	1841
Coles, Richard	Swanage	1797
Collier/Caler, Jane	Yeovil, Somerset	1820
Colmer, Nicholas	Milverton, Somerset	1786
Connock, Jane	unknown	1837
Cook, Sarah	Fordington	1817
Coombes, Miss Mary	Cerne Abbas	1783
Coombe/s	Beaminster	1815
Cooper, Isaac	Stoborough	1828
Cooper, Joseph	Stoborough	1828
Corben, William	Isle of Purbeck	1806
Cowan, Robert	Taunton, Somerset	1805
Cox, Joseph	Langport, Somerset	1786
Creech, Sarah	Dorchester	1839
Croade/Coade, Elizabeth	Preston	1812
Crocker, James	Bridport	1824
Curry, John	Chilton (Chilthorne Domer, Somerset?)	1816

Curtis, James	Cattistock	1832/1833
Curtis, Mary	Puddletown	1817
Dale, John	Blandford	1788
Darby, Mary	Bridport	1815
Darch, John	Bridgewater, Somerset	1784
Davey, George	Charmouth	1799
Davis , Ann	Hunsham/Huntsham, Devon	1786
Davis, Isabella [Billah]	South Petherton, Somerset	1825
Davis, Joseph Eggardon	Bradpole	1844
Davis, William	Haydon	1788
Davy, Elizabeth	Barrington, Somerset	1779
Day, Charles	Woolavington, Somerset	1805
Day, John	Purse Caundle	1804
Day, Joseph	Longburton	1819
Deacon/Dracon, Richard	Wanborough, Wiltshire	1815
Devenish, Isaac	Maiden Newton	1819
Dibben, Mary	Sturminster Newton	1835
Dowding, Eliza	Cerne Abbas	1844
Drake, Margaret	unknown	1779
Duck, Stephen	South Petherton, Somerset	1794
Dunford, Martha	Abbotsbury	1817
Eastment, John	Ryme Intrinseca	1839
Elkins, ?	Buckland Newton	1815
Elliott, Ann	South Petherton, Somerset	1804
Elliott, David	Beaminster	1842
Elliott, Wm	Martock, Somerset	1821
Ellis, Sarah	Cattistock	1810
Elward/Edward, William	Martock, Somerset	1800
England, Miss	South Petherton/Burrow Hill, Somerset	1809
England, Thomas?	Kingsbury, Somerset	1815
Evans/Ewens, John	Broadwindsor	1804
Evans, John	Yeovil, Somerset	1815
Farr/Fall, Wm	unknown	1845
Farr, John	Merriott, Somerset	1845
Fever, William	(Corton) Denham, Somerset	1783

Foot, William	Up Lyme, Devon	1785
Fortescue, William	Sherborne	1819
Foss, Joseph	Chideock	1829
Furmedge, Elizabeth	Corfe Castle	1790
Gander, Penelope	Sherborne	1794
Gape, John	unknown	1796
Gardener, John	Haselbury (Bryan, Dorset or Plucknett, Somerset)	1835
Gardener, Mary	Haselbury, Somerset	1815
Gaylard, Robert	Stoke under Ham, Somerset	1794
Gifford, Joseph	Hinton St George, Somerset	1798
Gifford, Sarah	unknown	1815
Gill, Joseph	Chard, Somerset	1787
Gould, Robert	Froome	1819
Grant, James	Exeter, Devon	1781
Grant, John	Exeter, Devon	1775
Gray, Sarah	Glastonbury, Somerset	1822
Grinton/Grinter, Phillis	Hinton St George, Somerset	1784
Grinton/Grinter, Rachael	Hinton St George, Somerset	1806
Gudge, Grace	Bridport, Dorset	1822
Gummer, Mrs	South Petherton, Somerset	1811
Guppy, Betty	Netherbury	1816
Guppy, Charles	Halstock	1779
Haines, John	Yetminster	1831
Hallett, Christian	Piddletrenthide	1817
Hansford, Robert	West Milton	1821
Harder, Joseph	Swanage	1812
Harding, Joseph	Purbeck	1813
Harrison, Esau	East Coker, Somerset	1834
Hart, Jane	Ansty	1796
Hawkins, Elizabeth	Weymouth	1818
Hawkins, Elizabeth	Abbotsbury	1817
Hawkins, James	Middlezoy, Somerset	1802
Hawkins, Mary Ann	Yeovil, Somerset	1826
Hawkins, Sarah	Stoughton Cross, Somerset	1807
Hawkins, Sarah	South Brent, Somerset	1809

Hawkins, Sarah	Weymouth	1817
Hawtry, Grace	Sherborne/Hackney, London	1830
Haynes, Elizabeth	Abbotsbury	1816
Hayward, Mary	Eggerton (Eggardon near Bridport)	1795
Helyar, Revd Henry	Hardington, Somerset	1831
Hill, John	Tarrant Launceston	1783
Hockey, Mary	Middle Chinnock, Somerset	1816
Hodder, Mary	St Peter's (Dorchester)	1840
Hodder, Mary	Plympton, Devon	1782
Hodges, Jane	Yeovil, Somerset	1810
Hole, George	Colyton, Devon	1785
Hood, John	Netherbury	1804
Hopkins, Samuel	Milton Abbas	1820
Horn, Philip	Wedmore, Somerset	1819
Hounsell, Nancy	Bridport	1781
Humphrey, Robert	Shipton Beauchamp, Somerset	1809
Hunt, George	Horsington, Somerset	1775
Hunt, Joseph	Hazelbury (Bryan)	1828
Hunt, Martha	Whitchurch	1814
Hutchings, John	Seavington St Mary, Somerset	1779
Ironside, Gilbert	Longbredy	1789
Jackson, Mrs	Axminster, Devon	1797
Jacob, John	Weymouth	1823
Jefferies/Jeffery, John	Haselbury (Plucknett), Somerset	1833
Jefford, Jane	Milton Abbas	1813
Jolliffe, Richard	Crewkerne, Somerset	1795
Joy, Walter	Wimborne, Dorset	1779
Keen, Philip	Mere, Wiltshire	1811
Kiddle, Samuel	Sydling St Nicholas	1842
King, Mrs	Sherborne	1801
King/Ring, Mark	Bradford (Abbas) or Compton (Nether or Over)	1819
Lamb, Susan Mayo/Mary	Bridport	1829
Langworthy, Mrs	Exeter, Devon	1800
Leach/Peach Douglas, Mrs	Clayton Street, Lambeth, London	1801

Lester, Elizabeth	Dorchester	1824
Lindquist, Amelia	Wyke Regis	before 1839
Lock, Henry	Chideock	1781
Lovell, Jane	Upwey	1839
Lover, Thomas	Hawkchurch	1816
Lucas, Uriah	Lettisham in Ditcheat, Somerset	1823
Major, George	Netherbury	1840
Mayo, George	Nether Compton	1818
Meech, William	Evershot	1800
Millard, Margaret	East Pennard, Somerset	1779
Monkhouse, Anna Elizabeth	Holwell, Somerset (Dorset from 1844)	1830
Moore, George	Sherborne	1840
Moore, Wm	unknown	1840
Muckle, Richard	Portland	1799
Mudford, Betty	East Coker, Somerset	1815
Mumford, Peter	Crewkerne, Somerset	1812
Nation, John	Exeter, Devon	1783
Newberry, Richard	Whimple, Devon	1775
Noake, Elizabeth	Broadwindsor	1817
Noake, Sarah	unknown	1802
Noake, Thomas	Milborne Port, Somerset or Purse Caundle, Dorset	1809
Norman, Henry	Winchester, Hampshire	1788
Oakes, Miss Betsy	London	1809
Pain, William	Netherhay in Broadwindsor	1840
Palmer, Joanna	Chardstock	1790
Palmer, Robert	Axminster, Devon	1794
Palmer, Thomas	Axminster, Devon	1812
Parker, Miss	Exeter, Devon	1795
Parker, Henry	Hutton/Hindon, Somerset	1809
Parker, Mr	Barton, Somerset	1825
Parker/Paster/Patience/Pashen, Elizabeth	Cerne Abbas	1830
Pearce, Elisha	Lyme, Regis	1843

Pearce, William	Mosterton	1830
Phelips, Edward	Montacute House, Somerset	1825
Phelips, Martha	Haselbury (Plucknett), Somerset	1825
Pierce, Wm	unknown	1833
Pinney, Pretor	Somerton House, Somerset	1809
Pinnock, Mary	Penzance, Cornwall	1811
Pitcher, William	Preston, Plucknett or Lyde, Yeovil, Somerset	1824
Pitfield, William Slade	Burton	1828
Pitt, James	Dewlish	1820
Pitt, Mary	Portland	1780
Pitts, Jane	Hazelbury (Plucknett), Somerset	1826
Poole, Susannah	Stalbridge	1782
Pople/Popler, William	Crewkerne, Somerset	1811
Pottle, Martin	Milborne St Andrew	1775
Prowse, Mary	South Petherton, Somerset	1806
Pummer, Thomas	Stalbridge, Dorset	1814
Redman, John	Edmonsham, Dorset	1798
Rendall/Randall, Elias	West Coker, Somerset	1822
Richards, John	Exeter, Devon	1790
Richards, William	Exeter, Devon	1791
Ross, James	Holwell, Somerset	1791
Samways, Ann	Walditch	1811
Scadding, James	Ilchester	1813
Scott, Susannah	North Curry, Somerset	1790
Sheppard, Richard	Maiden Newton	1813
Spear, Mary	Bere Regis	1803
Spong, John	Wimborne	1779
Shore, James	Haselbury, Somerset	1798
Standard, James	Whitchurch (Canonicorum)	1814
Stanton, Jane	Toller Porcorum	1843
Stephens, Jane	Dorchester	1805
Stephens, Jane	Weymouth	1809
Stevens, Jane Mrs	South Petherton, Somerset	1834
Stickland, Samuel	Meare (Mere, Wiltshire or Meare, Somerset)	1825

Stower, Hannah	Puckington, Somerset	1806
Strong, Sarah	Hatch, Somerset	1783
Stroud, Mary	Yetminster	1796
Sturmey, John	Langton, Dorset	1799
Swaffield, Charlotte	Corscombe	1815
Swaffield, Elizabeth	Weymouth	1842
Symes/Sims, Joseph	Bere Regis or 'Langton in Purbeck'	1816
Talbot, Patience	unknown	1836
Taverner, Thomas	unknown	1849
Taverner, William	Yeovil, Somerset	1817
Taylor, Edward	East Coker, Somerset	1804
Taylor, Elizabeth	Crewkerne, Somerset	1812
Thomas, John	Poxwell	1835
Thorne, Miss	Sherborne	1809
Thornhill, William	Portesham	1780
Toogood, Mrs	unknown	1835
Toogood, Robert	Motcombe	1802
Toogood, Robert	East Stower	1801
Tozer, George	unknown	1799
Travers, Jane	Bridport	1789
Tremlett, Ann	Exeter, Devon	1784
Trevitt, Richard	Puncknowle	1823
Tullidge, Elizabeth	Abbotsbury	1815
Tullidge, Mary	Dorchester	1815
Vickery, Elizabeth	Colyton, Devon	1790
Vors, Sarah Mrs	Chard, Somerset	1779
Vyvyan, Revd	Powerstock	1779
Warren, Job	Tincleton	1839
Webb, Jane	Netherbury	1814
Welch, James	Limington, Somerset	1815
Welch, James	West Cammel, Somerset	1814
Wellstead, Anne	Halstock	1844
Wellstead , James	Weymouth	1832
West, Jemima	Wedmore, Somerset	1819
Wheeler, Philip	Toller Porcorum	1812

White, John	Portland	1806
Whitmarsh, Elizabeth	Yeovil, Somerset	1843
Whitmarsh, Henry	Yeovil, Somerset	1842
Whitrow, Joseph	Kimmeridge	1815
Wilkins, Hannah	Yeovil, Somerset	1822
Wilkinson, Francis	Weymouth	1809
Willis, Mary	Puddletown	1815
Willmott, Mr	Beaminster	1802
Wills, Elizabeth	Isle Abbotts, Somerset	1797
Wills, George	Milborne Port, Somerset	1820
Wilmorton, William Highmore	Stafford in Barwick, Somerset	1819
Winter, Susannah	Bishops Lydiard, Somerset	1790
Withye, John	Sherborne	1844
Wood, Sarah	Dorchester	1783
Woolcott, Edward	Sidbury, Devon	1783
Woolfries, Thomas	Whatcombe in Winterborne Whitchurch	1780
Woolfry, John	Winterborne Whitchurch	1796
Woolley, Mrs	South Petherton, Somerset	1796
Young, George	Lymington, Somerset	1847
Young, Hannah	Cattistock	1831

Stockland patients		
Aplin, Amey	Chardstock, Devon	1831
Aplin, Elizabeth	unknown	1839
Aplin, Samuel	Coombe St Nicholas, Somerset	1829
Austin, Annie	unknown	1838
Bailey, John	Ottery St Mary	1838
Baker, Osmond	Pinhoe, Devon	1833
Baldwin, James	Barnstaple, Devon	1822
Batstone, Robert	Axminster, Devon	1840
Bennett, Jane	South Brent, Somerset	1830
Berry, Ann	Coombe St Nicholas, Somerset	1830
Bishop, Edmund	unknown	1838
Bond, Ann, D	Clyst Honiton, Devon	1832
Bowren/Bowring, Joel	Axminster, Devon	1828
Bowyer, Andrew	unknown	1834

Bridges, Sarah	unknown	1841
Brooke-Keat	unknown	1838
Broom, Grace	unknown	1835
Brown, Joseph	unknown	1835
Bucknell, Joseph	unknown	1836
Butter, Benjamin	unknown	1836
Chapman, Mary Ann	unknown	1839
Clapp, Robert	unknown	1840
Clarke, William	unknown	1838
Clatworthy, Grace	Seaton, Devon	1830
Cookney, Mary	unknown	1832
Crabb, Samuel	Pinhoe, Devon	1831
Cross, William	Axminster, Devon	1826
Dawe, Henry	Corscombe, Dorset	1838
Dean, Samuel	Chardstock, (Dorset to 1896 then Devon)	1820
Drake, Thomas	unknown	1838
Drewe, Jane	unknown	1832/33
Emmett, Hannah	Lyme Regis	1829
England, Joan	South Petherton, Somerset	1820
Eveleigh, Sarah	unknown	1835
Farrant, Mary	Axminster, Devon	1822
Ford, Mary	Cornwall[?]	1841
French, John	Kilmington, Devon	1830
German, Martha	Unknown –found wandering in Devon, brought from South Leigh, Devon	1830
Gillard/Gifford, Joseph	unknown	1834
Glyde, Eliza	Crewkerne, Somerset	1830
Good, Henry	unknown	1836
Gratten, James	Up Lyme, Devon	1830
Hamlett, John	unknown	1830
Hamlett, William	Thorncombe, Devon	1830
Hammett, Henry	Heavitree, Devon	1830
Hardy/Harding, James	Musbury, Devon	1829
Hart, Diana	unknown	1839
Harvey, Barrow	Banwell, Somerset	1825
Hayball, Thomas	Chard, Somerset	1825
Hitchcock, Ann	unknown	1833
Hitchcock, John	unknown	1834
Hitchcock, William	Thorncombe, Devon	1829
Honeybone, John	unknown	1833

Honeybull, John	unknown	1834
Honibond, William	unknown	1835
Honibone, Edward	unknown	1835
Huish, William	White Staunton, Somerset	1828
Hussey, Hannah	unknown	1837
Huxter, Joseph	unknown	1822
Johnson, Mary	Payhembury, Devon	1829
Kerby[?], Sarah	unknown	1836
Love, Mary/Nancy[?]	unknown	1834
Loveridge, Isaac	Lyme Regis	1829
Major, George	Netherbury	1831
Major, Samuel	Netherbury	1830
Marks, Robert	Axminster, Devon	1830
Merryweather, Mary	Charmouth, Dorset	1840
Miller, Sarah	unknown	1835
Mitchell, James	Sidbury, Devon	1830
Morey/Mooring, Robert	Chardstock, (Dorset to 1896 then Devon)	1840
Northcote, George	unknown	1837
Palmer, Ruth	Hawkchurch, Dorset	?/1829
Perris/Parris, Elizabeth	Colyton, Devon	1822
Perry, Mary	unknown	1833
Peters, William	Broadwindsor	1832
Phippen, Ruth	Thorncombe, Devon	1836
Pomeroy, George	Broadwindsor	1831
Poole, Elizabeth	unknown	1835
Pople, William	unknown	1835
Quick, John	Muddiford, Devon	1840
Reid, Elizabeth	unknown	1834
Roman, Susan	Lyme Regis	1833
Row, Henry	Musbury, Devon	1830
Sellers, Mary	Lyme Regis	1840
Shewbrook/Sholebrook, Samuel	unknown	1836
Sparks, Betty D	unknown	1832
Stukey, William J.	Winsham near Chard, Devon	1838
Symonds, Maria	unknown	1837
Thomas, Hannah	Honiton, Devon	1823
Thompson, Archibald	London	1832
Tolman, Peter	Chideock	1829
Tubb, William	unknown	1833
Turner, Elizabeth	unknown	1835

Vickary, Hannah	Seavington St Mary	1828
Wakely, Johana	Axminster, Devon	1837
Walters, Richard	Banwell, Somerset	1823
Webb, Eliza/Elizabeth	unknown	1834
Wheadon, William	Seaton, Devon	1828
Whitehead, J	Ottery St Mary	1841
Wilkins, John	unknown	1835
Wills, William	Seaton, Devon	1830
Wyatt, Benjamin	Upottery, Devon	1838
Unknown male	unknown	1833

APPENDIX 3

Diets in the asylums.

The issue of the diet of patients, particularly pauper patients, was raised by Visitors to all three of the Dorset asylums. The Axminster Union workhouse diet was presented by the Visitors to the asylum proprietor as a good basis for the diet at Stockland in 1837.[476]

However, despite efforts made by the Visitors it was reported six months later, in March 1838, that the change of diet had 'disagreed with the patients and that at present no regular system in this respect seems to be acted upon'. The subject was considered again in November 1839 when the Visitors 'interrogated some of the more intelligent patients separately with the view of ascertaining if they were properly taken care of'. The result of which was once again food related. However, during the same visit it was witnessed that the dinner appeared to be 'a sufficient meal with which they were satisfied'.

Axminster Union Workhouse, diet for able-bodied paupers, 1837.[477]
(see pages 228-229)

Transcript:

Breakfast	Men	Women	Children under 12
Every day	Bread - 7oz, milk broth 1.5 pints	Bread - 6oz, milk broth 1.25 pints	Bread - 6oz milk broth 1.25 pints

476   DHC, Q/A/L/Private/1.

477   TNA, MH 12/2095/293.

Dinner	Men	Women	Children under 12
Sunday, Wednesday and Friday	5oz meat,1lb potatoes,	4oz meat, 1.25lb potatoes,	3oz meat, 1lb potatoes
Monday	1lb potatoes, 10oz suet pudding	1.25lb potatoes, 8oz suet pudding	1lb potatoes, 6 or 8oz suet pudding
Tuesday, Thursday and Saturday	7oz potatoes. 1.5 pints soup	6oz potatoes. 1.25 pints soup	6oz potatoes. 1.25 pints soup

Supper	Men	Women	Children under 12
Everyday	7oz bread, 1.5 pints gruel or milk porridge, 2oz cheese	6oz bread,1 pint gruel or milk porridge, 1.5oz cheese	6oz bread, 0.5 pints gruel or milk porridge,1oz cheese

The Forston diet, 1838 and 1842.[478]
(see page 230)

The Forston diet was set out in the minute book of the visiting Justices of the Peace in 1838. It was the same for male and female patients and those engaged in active employment received unspecified 'extra diet':

Breakfast (everyday)	Milk porridge with 6oz bread
Dinner, 2 days each week	6oz cooked meat with vegetables
Dinner, 2 days each week	1lb suet or rice pudding
Dinner, 2 days each week	Soup with 6oz bread
Dinner, 1 day each week	Bread and cheese
Supper (everyday)	6oz bread, 2oz cheese, with ale.

By October 1842 the meals provided included five days of meat instead of four, one meal of soup having been withdrawn. This change had been well received and 'with good effect' on the health of the patients. The Visitor's reported that no increase in the maintenance fee was needed and remained at 7s. per week. A few months later the allowance of meat had doubled to almost 23oz per week.

478   DHC, NG-HH/CMR/2/1/2.

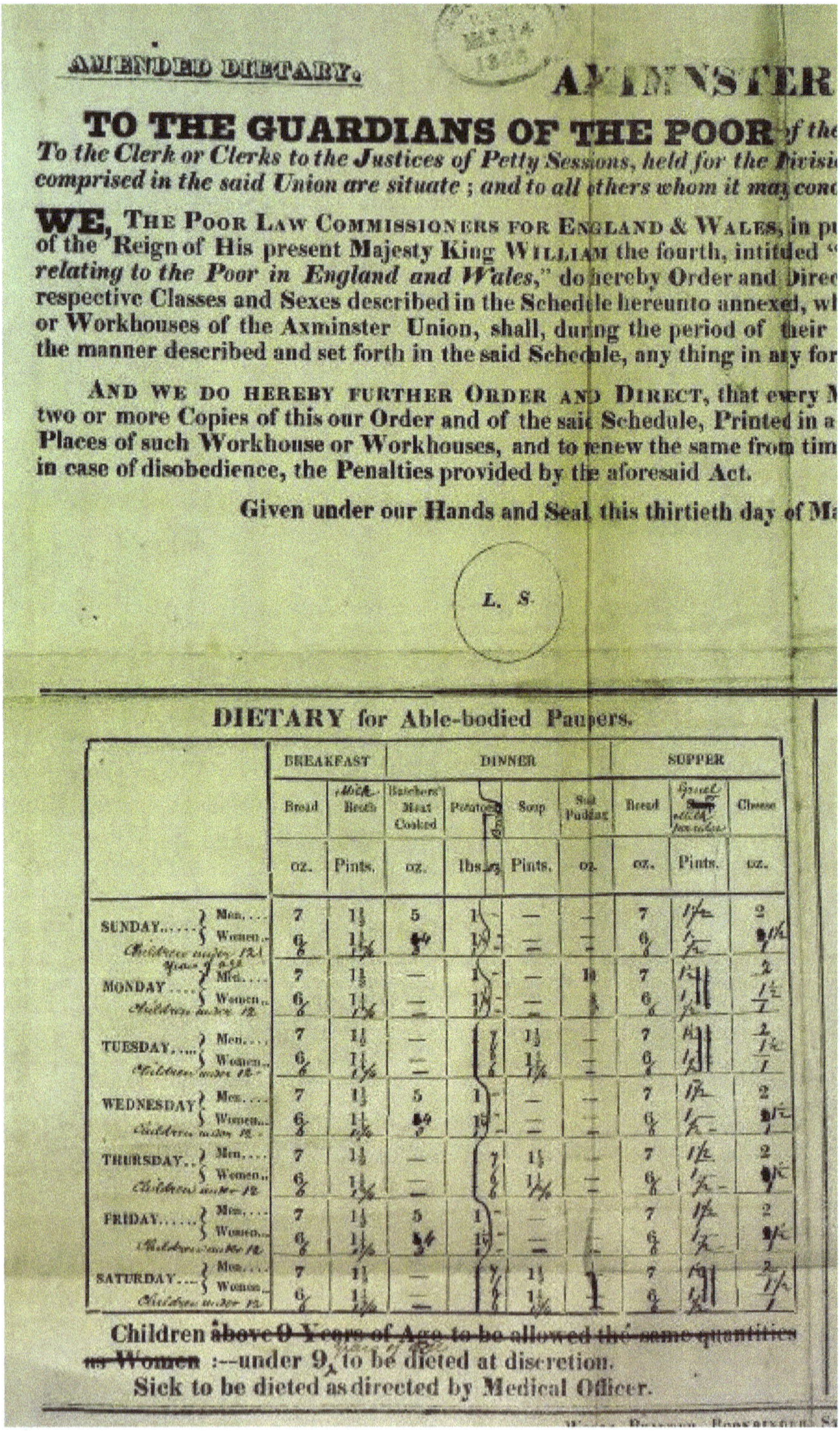

AMENDED DIETARY.

AXMINSTER

TO THE GUARDIANS OF THE POOR *of the*

To the Clerk or Clerks to the Justices of Petty Sessions, held for the Division comprised in the said Union are situate ; and to all others whom it may conc

WE, THE POOR LAW COMMISSIONERS FOR ENGLAND & WALES, in pu of the Reign of His present Majesty King WILLIAM the fourth, intituled " *relating to the Poor in England and Wales,*" do hereby Order and Direct respective Classes and Sexes described in the Schedule hereunto annexed, wh or Workhouses of the Axminster Union, shall, during the period of their the manner described and set forth in the said Schedule, any thing in any for

AND WE DO HEREBY FURTHER ORDER AND DIRECT, that every N two or more Copies of this our Order and of the said Schedule, Printed in a Places of such Workhouse or Workhouses, and to renew the same from tim in case of disobedience, the Penalties provided by the aforesaid Act.

Given under our Hands and Seal this thirtieth day of Ma

L. S.

DIETARY for Able-bodied Paupers.

		BREAKFAST		DINNER				SUPPER		
		Bread	Milk Broth	Butchers' Meat Cooked	Potatoes	Soup	Suet Pudding	Bread	Gruel or other liquid	Cheese
		oz.	Pints.	oz.	lbs.	Pints.	oz.	oz.	Pints.	oz.
SUNDAY	Men	7	1½	5	1	—	—	7	1½	2
	Women	6	1½	1½	1¼	—	—	6	1½	1½
	Children under 12 years of age									
MONDAY	Men	7	1½	—	1	—	10	7	1½	2
	Women	6	1½	—	1¼	—		6	1½	1½
	Children under 12									
TUESDAY	Men	7	1½	—	⅞	1½	—	7	1½	2
	Women	6	1½	—	¾	1½	—	6	1½	1½
	Children under 12									
WEDNESDAY	Men	7	1½	5	1	—	—	7	1½	2
	Women	6	1½	1½	1¼	—	—	6	1½	1½
	Children under 12									
THURSDAY	Men	7	1½	—	⅞	1½	—	7	1½	2
	Women	6	1½	—	¾	1½	—	6	1½	1½
	Children under 12									
FRIDAY	Men	7	1½	5	1	—	—	7	1½	2
	Women	6	1½	1½	1¼	—	—	6	1½	1½
	Children under 12									
SATURDAY	Men	7	1½	—	⅞	1½		7	1½	2
	Women	6	1½	—	¾	1½		6	1½	1½
	Children under 12									

Children above 9 Years of Age to be allowed the same quantities as Women :—under 9, to be dieted at discretion.
Sick to be dieted as directed by Medical Officer.

R UNION.

the AXMINSTER UNION, in the Counties of Devon and Dorset--
ision or Divisions of the said Counties in which the Parishes and Places
oncern.

pursuance of the Provisions of an Act passed in the fourth and fifth Years
d "*An Act for the Amendment and better Administration of the Laws*
rect that from and after the fifteenth day of June next the Paupers of the
who may now or hereafter be received and maintained in the Workhouse
ir residence therein, be fed, dieted, and maintained with the food and in
former Order to the contrary notwithstanding.

y Master of the Workhouse or Workhouses of the said Union, shall cause
n a legible manner and in a large type, to be hung up in the most public
ime to time, so that it be always kept fair and legible, on pain of incurring

May in the Year One Thousand Eight Hundred and Thirty-seven.

(*Signed*)

T. Frankland Lewis.
J. G. S. Lefevre.
Geo. Nicholls.

DIETARY for Aged and Infirm Paupers.

	BREAKFAST		DINNER				SUPPER		
	Tea	Bread	Butchers' Meat Cooked	Potatoes	Soup or Rice Milk	Rice or Suet Pudding	Bread	Cheese	Butter
		oz.	oz.	lbs	Pints	oz.	oz.	oz.	oz.
SUNDAY...............	One Pint daily or one Ounce in loft, and 7 ounces of Sugar weekly.	6	4	½	—	—	6	1	—
MONDAY...............		6	—	¾	—	10	6	1	—
TUESDAY...............		6	—	¾	1	—	6	—	½
WEDNESDAY...........		6	4	½	—	—	6	1	—
THURSDAY..........		6	—	1½	1	—	6	—	½
FRIDAY...............		6	4	½	—	—	6	1	—
SATURDAY...........		6	—	½	1	—	6	—	½

Four Ounces of Butter and one Pint of skimmed Milk per week.

Stationer, &c. Axminster.

DIETARY TABLE.

MALES.	FEMALES.
BREAKFAST.	**BREAKFAST.**
Milk, thickened with Oatmeal and Flour, 1 Pint. Bread, 6 ounces.	Milk, thickened with Oatmeal, and Flour, 1 Pint. Bread, 5 ounces.
DINNER.	**DINNER.**
Sunday, ... ⎤ Meat, 5 oz., cooked, Monday, .. ⎪ free from bone Wednesday, ⎬ and Thursday, .. ⎦ Vegetables. Tuesday, ... 1 Pint Soup, Bread 6 oz. Friday, ... 1 Pound Pudding. Saturday, ... Meat Pie Crust, 12 oz. Meat, 3 oz., Potatoes. Beer, Half a Pint daily.	Sunday, ... ⎤ Meat, 5 oz., cooked, Monday, .. ⎪ free from bone, Wednesday, ⎬ and Thursday, .. ⎦ Vegetables. Tuesday, .. 1 pint Soup, Bread, 5 oz. Friday, ... $\frac{3}{4}$lb Suet Pudding. Saturday, .. Meat Pie Crust, 12 oz. Meat, 3 oz., Potatoes. Beer, half a pint, daily.
SUPPER.	**SUPPER.**
Bread, 6 ounces, Cheese 2 ounces. Beer, half a pint.	Bread, 5 ounces, Butter, $\frac{1}{2}$ ounce. Tea, 1 pint.

The Out-door Workers and Laundry Women, have an extra quantity
of Beer, daily.

Forston diet, 1842

The Hanwell diet.[479]

Hanwell (Middlesex) was one of the asylums highlighted in the 1838 report which made various general and specific recommendations relating to improvement of institutions across the country. Hanwell's approach to patient care was progressive and alongside gentle employment it was believed that a nutritious diet aided recovery and was particularly beneficial to pauper patients. The proprietor at Stockland was 'cordially disposed' to act upon the Hanwell diet.

Like the Axminster Union diet there was no variation in breakfast

479   Ellis, *Treatise on the nature, symptoms, causes and treatment of insanity,* pp.340-1.

or supper. Dinner was a more varied meal. 'As the season affords' fruit pies might form an addition to the diet. Christmas was celebrated with roast beef and plum pudding and extras were allowed for sick patients.

One half-pint was allowed every day for those who were industrious and infirm. The healthy who did not work were not allowed malt liquor. Those who laboured out of doors, or who offered assistance in the wards, also received one third of a pint of beer at eleven in the morning and the same at four in the afternoon.

	Breakfast	Supper	Additional
Everyday	1.5 pint of rice or oatmeal gruel, as is deemed most conducive to health.	1.5 pint of rice or oatmeal gruel, as is deemed most conducive to health.	Bread - 14oz

	Dinner
Sunday	Roast beef, 6oz (in raw state), free from bone, 4oz yeast dumpling, 6oz vegetables. Sometimes potatoes substituted for dumplings.
Monday	Soup - made from meat boiled day before, with bones stewed, thickened with barley, rice, peas and vegetables, and flavoured with onions, pot-herbs and cayenne pepper.
Tuesday	As Sunday but with boiled mutton.
Wednesday	Soup - made from meat boiled day before, with bones stewed, thickened with barley, rice, peas and vegetables, and flavoured with onions, pot-herbs and cayenne pepper.
Thursday	Boiled pork
Friday	Soup - made from meat boiled day before, with bones stewed, thickened with barley, rice, peas and vegetables, and flavoured with onions, pot-herbs and cayenne pepper.
Saturday	14oz pie, made of coarse beef, with potatoes

APPENDIX 4

Terms used at Forston asylum to describe patients in 1841

	Males	Females
Mania	10	17
Mania with epilepsy	4	2
Mania with paralysis	2	
Melancholia	5	6
Melancholia with epilepsy		1
Melancholia with paralysis		1
Melancholia with occasional violence		6
Melancholia suicidal	1	2
Hypochondriasis		1
Incoherence	5	14
Incoherence with epilepsy		1
Incoherence with paralysis	1	
Incoherence with occasional violence	5	4
Incoherence suicidal		1
Imbecility	3	
Imbecility congenital		1
Dementia	10	2
Dementia with epilepsy	1	
Dementia with paralysis	1	
Idiocy	2	

Causes attributed for the condition of patients in the asylum, divided by the superintendent physician into categories of moral, physical and hereditary causes, 1841[480]

480   DHC, NG-HH/CMR/2/1/2.

Type of cause	Specific cause	Men	Women
		5	
Moral causes	Reverses (disengagement)		2
	Poverty	2	1
	Disappointed affections	2	8
	Domestic unhappiness	1	3
	Religious enthusiasm	2	1
	Grief		6
	Fright		7
Physical causes	Intemperance	4	1
	Injury of the head	4	1
	Mothers alarmed when pregnant	2	
	Typhus fever	1	
	Asthma	1	1
	Injury of the back	1	
	Congenital defect	5	3
	Childbirth		4
Hereditary disposition		11	14

APPENDIX 5

Public Acts of Parliament specifically relating to the treatment of lunatics, 1774-1900.

Additionally, Private Acts were passed relating to particular counties and asylums (none in Dorset) and legislation relating to workhouses, prisons, poor laws and local government included clauses relating to lunatics, idiots and insane persons.

1874 Madhouses Act (14 Geo.III, c.49)
1779 Madhouses Act (19 Geo.III, c.15)
1786 Madhouses Act 26 Geo.III, c.91)
1800 Criminal Lunatics Act (39 & 40 Geo.III, c.94)
1808 County Asylums Act (48 Geo.III, c.96)
1811 Marriage of Lunatics Act (51 Geo. III, c.79)
1815 County Asylums Amendment Act (55 George III, c.46)
1815 Criminal Lunatics Amendment Act (55 George III, c.117)
1819 Pauper Lunatics Act (59 George III, c.127)
1824 County Asylums Amendment Act (5 George IV, c.100)
1828 County Asylums Act (9 George IV, c.40)
1828 Madhouses Act (9 George IV, c.41)
1828 Chancery Lunatics Property Act (9 George IV, c.68)
1829 Madhouses Law Amendment Act (10 George IV, c.18)
1830 Property Act (4William IV, c.65) consolidated laws relating to infants, idiots, lunatics and people of unsound mind
1832 Madhouses Act (3 & 4 William IV, c.107)
1833 Chancery Lunatics Act (3 & 4 William IV, c.3)
1833 Madhouses Law Amendment Act (3 & 4 William IV, c.64)
1835 Madhouses Law Continuation Act (5 & 6 William IV, c.22)
1838 Madhouses Law Continuation Act (1 & 2 Victoria c.73)
1840 Insane Prisoners Act (3 & 4 Victoria c.54)
1841 Madhouses Law Continuation Act (5 Victoria c.4)
1842 Chancery Lunatics Act (5 & 6 Victoria c.84)
1842 Lunacy Inquiry Act (5 & 6 Victoria c. 87)
1845 Lunacy Act (8 & 9 Victoria c. 100)

1845 County Asylums Act (8 & 9 Victoria c. 126)
1846 County Asylums Amendment Act (9 & 10 Victoria c.84)
1847 County Asylums Amendment Act (10 & 11 Victoria c.43)
1852 Court of Chancery Act (15 & 16 Victoria c.87)
1853 Chancery Lunatics Act (16 & 17 Victoria c.70)
1853 Lunacy Amendment Act (16 & 17 Victoria c.96)
1860 Criminal Lunatics Asylums Act (23 & 24 Victoria c.75)
1862 Chancery Lunatics Act (25 & 26 Victoria c.86)
1862 Lunacy Amendment Act (25 & 26 Victoria c.111)
1882 Lunacy Regulation Amendment Act (45 & 46 Victoria c.82)
1883 Trial of Lunatics Act (45 & 46 Victoria c.38)
1884 Criminal Lunatics Act (47 & 48 Victoria c.6)
1885 Lunacy Act (48 & 49 Victoria c.52)
1886 Lunacy (Vacation of Seats) Act (49 & 50 Victoria c.16)
1886 Idiots Act (49 & 50 Victoria c.25)
1889 Lunatics Law Amendment Act (52 & 53 Victoria c.41)
1890 Lunacy Act (53 Victoria c.5)
1891 Lunacy Act (54 & 55 Victoria c.57)

BIBLIOGRAPHY

MANUSCRIPT SOURCES

Bristol Archives
P/St MR/R/3/11, Gloucester marriages, 1842-1844.

Devon Heritage Centre (DvnHC)
1215A/PR/1/2, Stockland parish, composite register, 1742-1812.
1215A/PR/1/2, Stockland parish, burial register, 1813-1858.

Dorset History Centre
BG-PL Records of Poole Poor Law Union.
D1/9661, Will of John Dennett, 1772.
D1/9732, Marriage settlement, Symes and Wiseman, 1729.
D-FFO/29/11, correspondence, J. T. Vining to J Mercer, 1846-1847.
D-RGB/KF/20, Abstract of deeds and papers relating to estates of Robert Larder, C.18th.
DC-BTB, Records of Bridport borough.
DC-LR, Records of Lyme Regis borough.
NG-HH/CMR, Records of Forston asylum and Herrison hospital.
NG-PB, Probate records.
NG-PR1/, Dorchester prison records.
PE-ABB, Records of Abbotsbury parish.
PE-ASH, Records of Ashmore parish.
PE-CDK, Records of Chideock parish.
PE-CMR, Records of Charminster parish.
PE-CRA, Records of Cranborne parish.
PE-HAL, Records of Halstock parish
PE-LR, Records of Lyme Regis parish.
PE-PUD, Records of Puddletown parish.
PE-WYK, Records of Wyke Regis parish.
Q/A/L/Criminal/1, Dorset Quarter Sessions, criminal lunatics, correspondence, 1831-1843.
Q/A/L/Criminal/2, Dorset Quarter Sessions, criminal lunatics, prisoner files, 1877-1878.
Q/A/L/Private/1, Dorset Quarter Sessions, private mental health patients, registers.

Q/A/L/Private/2, Dorset Quarter Sessions, private mental health patients, plans.
Q/A/L/Private/3, Dorset Quarter Sessions, private mental health patients, certificates.
Q/D/E(L)/4/24/12, Dorset Quarter Sessions, land tax (Wambrook), 1812.
Q/D/E(L), Dorset Quarter Sessions, land tax.
Q/D/L(V), Dorset Quarter Sessions, alehouse licences.
Q/S/J, Dorset Quarter Sessions, jury lists.
Q/S/M, Dorset Quarter Sessions, minute and plea books.
T/CRA, Cranborne tithe map and apportionment, 1844-1847.
T/HAL, Halstock tithe map and apportionment, 1844-1846.

Somerset Heritage Centre
D/P/CHARD, Records of Chard parish.
D/P/WAM, Records of Wambrook parish.
D/P/CHI.DOM, Records of Chilthorne Domer parish.

The National Archives
HO 13 Criminal entry books, 1782-1871.
HO 17 Criminal petitions, 1819-1866.
HO 27 Criminal petitions, 1805-1892.
IR 1 (volume 21), Register of stamp duties, apprentices, 1710-1811.
IR 29/10/199, Stockland tithe map and apportionment, 1844.
MH 12/2095/293, Axminster poor law union, correspondence relating to workhouse diets, 1838.
MH 12/2096/253, Axminster poor law union, extracts from the minutes of the board of guardians, 1842.
MH 94/7, Lunacy Commission & Board of Control, patients admission register, 1846-1921.
PCOM 2/418, Winchester Gaol: calendar of trials at Assizes for the County of Southampton, 1816-1853.
PCOM 2/421, Winchester Gaol, Hampshire: calendar of trials at Quarter Sessions for the County of Southampton, 1829-1840.

Wiltshire and Swindon History Centre
1160/3, Great Wishford parish, composite register, 1538-1812.
A1/560/3, Old Manor formerly Fisherton House, Fisherton Anger, Register of Admissions, with minutes of Visitors, 1813-1868.
D1/62/4, Marriage licence bonds, 1628-1841.
P16/255, Will of Edward Symes, 1730.
P5/1750/25, Will of Thomas Mercer, 1750.

Wimborne St Giles, Lord Shaftesbury's archive
SE/P/39, Report of select committee on lunatics, with proceedings of committee, minutes and evidence, 11 Apr. 1859; with manuscript notes made by the earl of Shaftesbury to 1877.
LE, Leases of property

REPORTS OF GOVERNMENT COMMITTEES

'Report from the Select Committee on the State of Lunatics, Part 1 Original Communications, April 1808', *The Edinburgh Medical & Surgical Journal*, volume 4, pp.129-144.

Report together with the minutes of evidence from the select committee appointed to consider the provision being made for the better regulation of private madhouses in England, (ed.) J. Sharpe, (London, 1815).

Report of the Metropolitan Commissioners in Lunacy to the Lord Chancellor: presented to both houses of Parliament by command of Her Majesty / [by the Earl of Shaftesbury], (London, 1844).

MONOGRAPHS, THESES AND JOURNAL ARTICLES

Blackstone, W., *Commentaries on the Laws of England*, (Oxford, 1765-1769).

Brown, J. M., *A History of Dorset Hospitals* (PHD Thesis, Bristol University, 1967).

Burke, B., 'Richard Sheridan', *A genealogical and heraldic history of the landed gentry of Great Britain & Ireland*, volume 2, (London, 1879).

Ellis, W. C., *A Treatise on the Nature, Symptoms, Causes and Treatment of Insanity with Practical Observations on Lunatic Asylums and A Description of the Pauper Lunatic Asylum for the County of Middlesex at Hanwell*, (London, 1838).

Fisher, D. R., 'Seymour Edward Adolphus, Lord Seymour (1804-1885)', *History of Parliament* (2009).

Holloway, S. W. F. 'The apothecaries act, a reinterpretation', *Medical History*, volume 10 (1966), 107-129.

Hutchins, J., *The History & Antiquities of the County of Dorset*, 3rd Edition, 4 volumes (London, 1861-1874).

Jones, K., *Lunacy, Law and Conscience, 1744-1845* (Abingdon, 1955).

Lemmey, P., Smith J. and Stephenson, Y., *The Story of St Mary's Halstock*, (Bridport, 2009).

Levene, A., 'Parish apprenticeship and the old poor law in London', *Economic History Review*, 63 (2010), 915-41.

Newman, R., 'Laverstock house asylum', *Laverstock and Ford, chapters from local history*, Sarum Chronicle Sarum Studies, volume 6 (2019).

Parry-Jones, W. Ll, *The Trade in Lunacy* (Abingdon, 1972).

Parry-Jones, W. Ll., 'English Private Madhouses in the Eighteenth and Nineteenth Centuries', *Journal of the Royal Society of Medicine*, volume 66 (1973), pp.23-8.

Ritch, A., 'Workhouse or asylum? Accommodating pauper lunatics in nineteenth-century England', *Medical History*, volume 67 (2023), pp.109–127.

Rogers, J. (ed.), *In the Course of Time - A History of Herrison Hospital and Mental Health Care in Dorset (1832 -1992)*, (West Dorset Mental Health NHS Trust, 1992).

Shelford, L., *Definition of Sound and Unsound Mind, Chapter III, Practical Treatise of the Law, concerning Lunatics, Idiots and Persons of Unsound Mind* (London, 1847).

Tempel, M. van der, Wouters, I., Descamps F. and Aerts, D., *Ventilation techniques in the 19th century: learning from the past.* (Vrije Universiteit Brussel, Belgium, 2011).

Thorne, R. G., 'Browne, Francis John, 1754-1863, of Frampton', *History of Parliament* (1986).

Thorne, R. G., 'Gordon, Robert, 1786-1864, of Leweston House nr Sherborne', *The History of Parliament* (1986).

Tuke, S., *Description of the Retreat, an institution near York for insane persons of the Society of Friends* (London, 1813).

WEBSITES

Devon County Mental Hospital, social attitudes and mental illness in Devon 1845-1987, https://dcmh.exeter.ac.uk/

Eikelmann, C., *The Mountravers Plantation Community,* 1734-1834, https://seis.bristol.ac.uk/~emceee/mountraversplantationcommunity.html

Royal College of Surgeons of England, *Plarr's Lives of the Fellows,* https://livesonline.rcseng.ac.uk

A vision of Britain through time, https://www.visionofbritain.org.uk/

INDEX

www.ingramcontent.com/pod-product-compliance
Lightning Source LLC
Chambersburg PA
CBHW071736270326
41928CB00013B/2703